Praise for *Seeking Peace*

"This warm, wonderful book is loaded with ideas and insights to help you let go of your difficulties and obstacles and become everything you are meant to be."
— Brian Tracy - Author, Speaker, Consultant

"As I read Dr. Tan's *Seeking Peace*," I felt it was a road map of my own life. A roadmap that I had discovered in parts and pieces, discovered while falling on my face over and over again. There I found the roadmap and the lifelines that made me sustain my sanity and be able to thrive at the same time. The proven 5 fingers method makes the road clearer and the horizon peaceful.

"Dr. Birgitte Tan's philosophy is amazingly simplified, practical, and human friendly. Her thoughts are deeply rooted into fertile soils of our society. Soils that are rich with "Human Vitamins". *Seeking Peace* is the tree that Dr. Tan cultivated in her despair and even during the dark valley of her life. Its fruits will be abundant. It will nourish members of planet Earth. Their lives will be fearless and their love for one another will become unconditional."
— Dr. George Apelian

"*Seeking Peace* is a quick, easy-to-read insightful book. Dr. Tan's real-life examples of tragedies throughout the book are easily relatable. I'm in awe that her tools for thriving under difficult situations are actually simple and easy to follow. When you are going through a difficult time mentally and emotionally, complex methods are not what you need. Dr. Tan's book gives tools of hope that you can use to cope through tragedies in an effortless and positive way."
— Nida Padilla, Program Manager, Cancer Support Community Redondo Beach

"This book has a lot of gold nuggets in here that I'm sure will help a lot of people. I'm so inspired. What a great example of endeavoring and stepping into your greatness."

— Lois Blumenthal, TV Editor & Filmmaker

"Significant loss or change in your life drops you into a maze of the unknown. In this maze of difficult feelings, it is essential to have a guide to understand how to navigate it, because often the pain and discomfort will only send you deeper into the maze. *Seeking Peace* is that guide! There is often a disconnect between how we feel and how our intellect tries to make sense of it. In this book, you are given the tools to understand the true root of the pain and disorienting emotions you are feeling. It frames Dr. Tan's years of experience in successfully managing change in people's lives into clear pictures and strategies that help you create meaning and action that will serve you living a life of thriving. As a primary care doctor, a life coach, and a person who has felt the pain of change, *Seeking Peace* has helped me to heal myself, and others, in completing the emotions of loss and change, in pulling myself out of the maze and back on the path of living a life I love."

— Chris Yee, MD, Transformative Coaching, Life Abundant Consulting

"Author Dr. Birgitte Tan has written a hugely helpful book. *Seeking Peace* is a must-read for anyone going through tough times. This easy to read book provides you with simple skills and highly effective tools that will guide you in exactly how you can thrive through any adversity and, ultimately, come out a winner."

— Mary Morrissey, Founder of Brave Thinking Institute

SEEKING PEACE

The Proven 5-Fingers Method to THRIVE
Through Change Effortlessly

Dr. Birgitte Tan

Seeking Peace: The Proven 5-Fingers Method to THRIVE Through Change Effortlessly

www.FromGrievingToJoyfulLiving.com

Copyright © 2020 by Dr. Birgitte Tan

Published by Dance Away Sadness Publishing
Thousand Oaks, CA 91362

100% of the proceeds from the sale of this book will be donated to the International Childhood Cancer Charity, a 501(c)(3) organization.

Author services by Pedernales Publishing, LLC.
www.pedernalespublishing.com

Front cover design: Brittany Rockwell

Library of Congress Control Number: 2019914946

ISBN 978-0-578-58298-6

Printed in the United States of America

DEDICATION

This book is dedicated to my parents, Tanamas Hartanto and Helenna Jahja, and to my mentor and spiritual mother, Mary Morrissey.

Thank you Mom and Dad for bringing me into this world and providing me with the best life and opportunities. Your love brought me into this world and your love keeps me going through all the tough times. Thank you for your never-ending love and support.

Thank you Mary Morrissey for teaching me the essentials tools and skills to transform my tragedies into triumphs and how to share this gift with others who need it. Thank you for helping me continue to become a better version of myself.

I love you all very much. Thank You!

With utmost love and gratitude,
Birgitte Tan

ACKNOWLEDGMENTS

This 5-Fingers Method was inspired by the "5-finger rules for having a great day" by the late Reverend Jack Boland. Rev. Boland was a mentor of my mentor, Mary Morrissey. Even though I have never met Rev. Boland personally, his wisdom and teachings continue to bring light to many of us. I am grateful and honored to be able to learn from and further share the wisdom and teachings from Rev. Boland and Mary Morrissey.

CONTENTS

Dedication...iv

Acknowledgements vii

Introduction: Why the 5-Fingers Method? 1

Chapter 1: Two-Thumbs-Up Tears...................................7
   Love After the Inferno 7
   Acknowledge, Honor, and Let Go...........................10
      Acknowledge and Treat Your Abscess.................10
      Honoring the Horrible 12
      Let Go of Resistance.......................................13
   Let Them Flow, Let Them Flow, Let the Tears Flow 14
      The Body Knows...15
      Crying is Being Strong 17
      Dry Glue...18
   Midnight Thumbs-Up 20
      Don't Stay Over 21
      Was Cinderella Lucky?.....................................22
      Choose "Two Thumbs Up" NOW.......................23
   Beautifully Imperfect 24
   Review...26

Chapter 2: Chameleon Fingerprint...................................27
   Chameleon 28
      Loveless Honeymoon.......................................28
      The Retirement Trap 32

Explosive Edith..35
Eighteen Scars of Shame 37
The Yogis and Einstein..................................41
The Shape-Shifting Chameleon......................42
Fingerprint 44
    Lost in the Stage 44
    No Resuscitation......................................46
    Roscoe 48
    Heart with Ears on Open Hands 49
Review..52

Chapter 3: Muddled in the Middle 55
Un-Muddling the Misunderstanding...............56
    Not a Broken Loser..................................56
    You Are Whole and Courageous 58
    Time Does Not Heal All 59
    Staying Busy Does Not Allow Healing........60
    Running or Hiding is Futile 62
    The Turmoil of Thoughts 63
    Hung by a String of Gs 66
    The "F" Word...69
New Beginning...71
    Forget-Me-Not...71
    No Spiritual Bypass..................................73
Review..75

Chapter 4: Forward-Fortitude 77
The Sky Falls Again 78
    A Date at the MRI 78
    Hopes Unmet 85
Forward-Fortitude...88
    Is the Beach Ball Red or Green?................88
    The Nine-Second Master Move 90
    Breathe in the Simple Present..................93
    NATO with Gratitude 97

Circle of Laughter 102
Painting and Marching in Bubble Bath 105
Let's "Cheers" 111
Review 112

Chapter 5: Little Butterfly 115
Little Seed of Golden Green Plum 115
Little Messy Butterfly and Phoenix 121
Lighten Up 126
The Little Ant That Could 127
Closing Words 128
Wabi-Sabi Dream 128
To Do or Not to Do: It Is Your Choice 130
Review 131

References 133

Appendix 135

Disclaimer and Crisis Lines 143

Contact Information and Additional Resources 145

About ICCC (International Childhood Cancer Charity) ..147

INTRODUCTION

WHY THE 5-FINGERS METHOD?

Changes and losses are unavoidable as we go through adulthood. The question is not whether we are going to experience a tough time at some point in our lives, but how we can experience a tough time and still have peace of mind. How can we move effortlessly beyond our tragedy, rediscover joy, and thrive? The 5-Fingers Method will help ease our painful journey toward healing even after our lives seemingly fall apart.

I was living a beautiful, perfect life for over forty years until one night it all came crashing down. On that fateful October night, my former husband, seemingly out of the blue, declared that he no longer wanted to be married, and I watched him move out of our home. It was a month before our fifteenth wedding anniversary. It left me in great shock. I was so confused, sad, and scared.

As if the abrupt ending of my marriage wasn't enough pain and shock, life kept throwing more rotten lemons at me over the next two years. I lost my relationship with my family (who blamed me for the divorce), one of my cats died, I lost a significant amount of money, and my mother had a nervous breakdown because of the stress and shame of my divorce. Before I even had a chance to recover from these tragic events, I got diagnosed with cancer, my best friend and guardian angel died suddenly, and my last remaining cat died nine days after my best friend's passing. Each time a disastrous event happened, the pain and shock that ran through me was increasingly devastating, and hopelessness became my watchword.

I felt like I had been hit by an earthquake, swept away by a tornado, and then thrown into a deep lake of fire, and I had no idea how I would find the strength to go on another day. At times, I wished that I could just die and leave this world. But I didn't die. Instead, I grasped at every branch to keep me afloat. I knew I needed to stay strong at whatever cost, but I didn't know how to do it.

Eight years later, my life was beautiful once again. Through trial and error of techniques I gleaned from multiple books and programs, I not only survived my tragedies, I learned to evolve and thrive in my new life. Eight years after that fateful night, I found myself living a joyful, healthy, abundant life; that was, until I woke up one morning to find that a couple of fingers on my right hand were not moving with the rest. Within two weeks from this dark morning, I lost the strength, control, and function of all the fingers on my dominant right hand, followed by the entire hand and arm, limiting my ability to perform my job. Exhaustive, costly specialist consultations and tests could not successfully find the cause of the problem, and therefore no treatment was possible.

I had become handicapped within two weeks and was at risk of losing my job. All of a sudden, my financial stability, my future, and my ability (as the only child) to take care of my aging parents were all in jeopardy. My world was unexpectedly crumbling again. Before I had the time to fully adjust to my new handicap, my mother suddenly fell very ill. A myriad of diagnostic tests were unable to determine the cause of her illness, and she continued to suffer. Even worse than my own strange ailment was watching helplessly as my mother continued to suffer. As if these emotional and physical disasters were not enough, a couple of months later, my relationship with my boyfriend of seven years ended. He had been the one by my side as I recovered and rebuilt my life. Even though it was a mutual agreement between both of us and we still remain good friends, I felt that my heart was broken and bleeding again.

I felt as if life hit me hard and shattered me into little pieces, again. However, I avoided the same agony, anguish, and despair that I had experienced eight years ago. Yes, I was sad for the loss of my romantic relationship. Yes, I was concerned for my mother's health. However, this time I experienced the sadness and uncertainty with calmness and peace of mind. This time I did not have to go through the emotional turmoil of my tragedies, even in light of losing my dear mother, my ability to continue working in a field in which I had invested twenty-five years, and my most important confidante. I realized that the reason for my peace of mind this time, despite the tragedies, was that I had mastered the skills and tools for navigating my emotions with more ease and grace.

We are all going to experience changes in this life. As adults, we will have to go through tough times and triumph over the accompanying grief. Grief comes not only with death, divorce, or dire diagnosis. Grief, according to The Grief Recovery Institute®, "is the conflicting feelings caused by a change in our familiar routine." Life is full of changes. Loss is inevitable if we live our lives through adulthood, whether it is the loss of a relationship, a loved one, a dear pet, personal safety, or even loss of health or hope. We, or someone we care for, may become very ill. Community shootings may occur near us and rattle our lives even if we don't lose any family members or friends in the shooting. Our relationships end. People betray us. Our hopes and dreams don't come true. All these events in our lives can cause grief. And yet, most of us never learn how to effortlessly move through—and beyond— our tough times and the associated grief.

I have compiled these essential tools for navigating through tough times and grief with ease so you can have less agony and anguish as you go through your dark night. Each of these mental tools and skills are reflected onto each of our five fingers to make it easier for us to remember them and apply them where appropriate. I hope that this simple yet proven 5-fingers tool will help you not only to survive, but to move effortlessly through your emotional and physical tragedies and heal quickly from your grief. I want you to thrive.

I wish you all the best and hope you thrive with more ease, grace, fun, and joy.

> With love and gratitude
> from my heart to yours,
> Birgitte

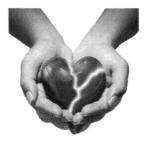

Chapter 1

TWO THUMBS UP TEARS

T he first step for navigating through disaster comes from our thumb. Embracing a "two thumbs up" attitude with a positive outlook while still acknowledging the grief that comes along with our disaster and allowing our tears to flow will help us to stay strong and move through our tragedy with more ease and grace.

LOVE AFTER THE INFERNO

My phone rang and I answered. "Hi, thank you for calling. This is Birgitte Tan. How may I help you?" A distressed male voice replied, "Hi, I'm Mark. I was looking for help for victims of the recent Santa Rosa fire, and I saw your post online saying that you are providing a free grief class for people who lost their homes in the fire. Is that correct?"

"Yes," I replied. "I am offering the 'Staying Strong While Your World is Burning' class for free to people who have been affected by the fire. Thank you for reaching out to me. How can I help you?"

Mark then told me that he and his sister, Ellen, had both lost their homes in the fire. Now that they were both safe in a temporary facility, Mark had been relentlessly looking for resources and support to help himself and his sister recover. He told me it had been tough trying to get back on his feet, and he was very concerned about his sister too.

"Ellen has turned into a hermit since the fire," Mark said. "She set up a camp on the grounds of her property and refuses to talk to anyone. I've been letting her know every time I find free help to rebuild our homes, but she thinks people will take advantage of her somehow. You sound patient and sincere. Can you talk to her if I can get her on the phone? I must warn you that she can be harsh with her words."

I assured Mark, "Yes, I am happy to talk to Ellen, and I will not be offended by anything she might say. Is she safe? Is she suicidal?"

I never did speak with Ellen, who thankfully was not suicidal, but continued to resist anyone's offer to help her. Mark took the "Staying Strong While Your World is Burning" class on his own; it helped him to navigate and resolve his own grief, and to better support his sister.

A year passed, and Mark called me with updates. He was rebuilding his home and doing well emotionally. "Occasionally I am still sad that the old house burned down, but I am rebuilding a new home the way I always wanted—with more bathrooms, windows, and a bigger master bedroom. Oh, and I met a wonderful lady who also lost her house, and we are close friends now—*very* close friends, you know." He chuckled a little and continued, "As you taught us, there is a seed of greater good in every adversity. It was such a horrible experience, but I'm grateful I learned the skills to recover, and I know I'll be just fine."

I congratulated Mark and told him that I was well pleased and very proud of him. "And how's your sister Ellen doing?" I asked.

Mark's voice changed: "She makes me sad. She is so suspicious of everybody and so negative that it's tiring to be around her. She is living in a shack that she built on her property. She'll never be able to recover and rebuild if she won't let anyone help her. And now she's upset at me because I'm moving on and she is not, but she chooses to be stuck. I'm so glad I chose to focus on the possible good. Even now, it's already great, and I know it will become even better if I stay positive, keep focusing on the possible good, and take one step at a time to rebuild." Even though we were talking on the phone, I could hear the smile in Mark's voice.

ACKNOWLEDGE, HONOR, AND LET GO

The first thing we want to do when changes happen that bring us grief is to acknowledge and honor them, instead of denying or trying to run away from them. It is instinctive for us to want to move away from something that is unpleasant, but trying to hide from grief will only cause more problems in the long run.

Acknowledge and Treat Your Abscess

Imagine that you wake up with sharp pain inside of your belly the day before you are supposed to go out of town for a very important work trip. You go to the doctor, and a few hours later, you're told that you seem to have somehow swallowed a sliver of bone that is now lodged in your intestine. It has led to an infection, and an abscess is forming inside your belly, so you need surgery tomorrow. Would you go into denial and pretend that you were not in pain? Would you decide to ignore your infected intestine and go on the work trip?

If you ignore or deny an abscess, it is very likely that the infection will get even worse and lead to sepsis, which is a widespread infection throughout the whole body. By the time sepsis occurs, the infection will have grown worse than you can imagine. It will have spread to all the organs in the body, affecting their functions and leading to organ failure that will eventually kill you. It is a lot easier to treat an abscess than to treat sepsis. We want to acknowledge and treat our abscess before it becomes a stealthy, widespread infection.

Experiencing the grief of an emotional disaster is like having an abscess in our intestines. If we ignore our grief, it will get worse. At first, the inflammation from the trauma causes severe pain. Over time, our grief will start to affect our entire system, just like sepsis. Denying our grief, whether that means trying to ignore it, numbing ourselves to it, or "toughing it out," will only cause the pain to continue. Unresolved grief will influence our peace of mind, affect our ability to sleep, and eventually manifest itself in physical symptoms. Unresolved grief will also impair our judgment and our ability to experience love and joy in our lives.

One common example of unresolved grief affecting our judgment is when there has been a betrayal in a relationship. If someone we love or trust has betrayed us, the unresolved grief from this emotional trauma could cause us to be afraid of getting hurt again, fearful that the next person might also betray us. We often become overly protective of ourselves. We might become very suspicious and overreact when things are not as perfect as we expect them to be. We imagine the worst when, for instance, our potential new partner needs to reschedule a date, and thus we make a judgment based on fear instead of love. We might also subconsciously keep our potential new true love at arm's length, which eventually leads to a lonely, loveless life. Trying to push grief away instead of healing our heart completely will bring more pain.

We cannot leave an infected abscess buried inside of our bodies. The inflammation will continue to discharge pus, causing more pressure and more pain until eventually the abscess ruptures once the damaged tissue cannot contain it anymore.

When we keep burying our grief, it likewise will cause more internal pressure on our emotional states that will, sooner or later, "explode." We will say and do things that we don't mean, usually in a very untimely manner. According to the Grief Recovery Method, an evidence-based grief recovery program, "Grief is cumulative and cumulatively destructive." If left unresolved, it will affect our lives in more ways than we can imagine. We need to face the challenge in order to resolve it. When it is an emotional challenge, the only way to fully heal is by acknowledging and allowing ourselves to feel it. What we want to do is acknowledge that we have been hurt and take the steps to heal.

Honoring the Horrible

Now that we understand the power and stealth of grief, we want to honor it. Merriam-Webster.com defines honor as "regard with great respect." When we experience an emotional disaster, we want to honor the grief associated with it. Just as when we interact with a person who can affect our life significantly, we want to interact with our grief promptly, mindfully, carefully, and smartly.

Having grief come into our life is as if the police were standing at our door with a warrant, demanding to interview us regarding something that we know we are utterly innocent of. We would be much better off going through the interview than slamming the door on the police. Even if we want to have our attorney present, we politely tell the police that we are calling our attorney first. We do not make the police stand at our door while we do our laundry and mow our lawn; we need to deal with them promptly in order to be able to move on with our lives.

Having grief is like having the police at our front door. As much as we would prefer they were not there, we need to treat them with respect as soon as we can. Our grief can afflict our lives in more ways than the police with a warrant can. Acknowledge and honor the grief, treat it with respect, and immediately give it the space and attention it deserves. This way, we will be in a much better mental and physical state in the long run.

Let Go of Resistance

What we resist, persists. Have you ever tried to complete a task that you disliked but still had to do? We all have, at one point or another. It is natural for us to resist what we don't want in our lives. Yet, the more resistance we have toward doing this task, the more unpleasant and challenging it gets. Resisting our feelings and grief when a disaster strikes us is like refusing to wash the dirty dishes piling up in the kitchen sink. The longer we leave it, the more caked the food residue will be on the plates, sometimes to the point of staining the dishes (even after we eventually wash them). If we continue to ignore our pile of dirty dishes, very soon they will start to smell, thereby ruining our kitchen, home, and life even more.

The problem is, unlike with dirty dishes, we cannot just throw away our lives. We each have only one life to live, so when we are faced with an emotional disaster, let's acknowledge the grief and let go of the resistance. Resisting our grief is another manifestation of trying to push away or deny our trouble, which we already know can lead to worse consequences. We want to accept the fact that grief has happened and promptly navigate through it as best we can so that we can move on faster and thrive after our tragedy.

LET THEM FLOW, LET THEM FLOW, LET THE TEARS FLOW

I walked into our office and found our oncologist sitting at her desk, facing the wall in tears. I had never seen her cry in the seven years we had worked together.

"Are you okay? What's wrong?" I asked.

She ducked her head down and said, "I'm sorry I'm crying. My dad just had a heart attack. He is in the ICU now. I'm so scared. My mom died three years ago from a heart attack, and I never got over it." She looked up at me with tears still streaming down her face and swallowed hard. "I'm sorry I'm crying like this. I'll stop in a minute." She swallowed hard again, clenched her jaws and her fists, and shook her head as if to shake off any feelings she might have. "I'll be fine. Sorry you have to see me crying like a baby; sorry I'm such a wimp."

"You are not a wimp at all. It is good to cry when we have a traumatic experience," I said to her quietly.

"Well, it wasn't like I was struck by a bolt of lightning and broke my legs. Sorry for being a big crybaby," she replied.

"Not physically, but in a way, metaphorically, you were struck by a bolt of lightning that broke your heart, again. And just as it is normal and good to cry from physical pain, it is normal and good to cry from emotional pain. Even our bodies produce emotional tears, in addition to our basal and reflex tears."[2]

The oncologist gave me a quizzical look. "There are three different tears?"

"Yes," I replied. "There are emotional, basal, and reflex tears."

The Body Knows

"Our reflex tears contain mostly water and are released as a response to physical irritants such as dust or wind.[2] Our basal tears are a protein-rich antibacterial liquid that our bodies constantly release for the sole purpose of lubricating and protecting our eyes.[2] Our emotional tears, on the other hand, contain substances such as prolactin, adrenocorticotropic hormones, and leucine-enkephalin, all of which are released to help us cope with the stress from our grief.[2] Emotional tears are released when we cry out of sadness, fear, pain, anguish, or anxiety.[2]

"Studies have shown that the release of emotional tears affects our bodies differently than reflex or basal tears.[3,4] Our emotional tears help reduce pain and help us tolerate stress better. The leucine-enkephalin in our emotional tears is an endorphin that reduces pain and improves our mood; it is our bodies' natural opioid. The adrenocorticotropic hormone has a vast array of functions, including the regulation of blood pressure and blood sugar. It is anti-inflammatory, and it is important for helping our bodies to tolerate stress. Prolactin is commonly known as the lactation hormone; however, this hormone also contributes to our ability to respond to stress, mount an appropriate immune response, and regulate our emotions.

"In addition to releasing these three hormones, when we cry out of sadness, fear, pain, or anxiety, our bodies also release oxytocin—a neurotransmitter and a hormone that is released in our hypothalamus during childbirth, sex, and lactation.[3] It is known as the nurture or love hormone because it also reduces anxiety, cardiac stress, and depression. Lastly, emotional crying further activates our parasympathetic nervous system.[3] As opposed to the sympathetic nervous system (which induces our fight-or-flight response), our parasympathetic nervous system, when activated, decreases our heart rate and blood pressure, thus helping us to calm down. All these changes that occur in our bodies tell us that crying is a natural, normal, and beneficial process when we are in distress, emotionally and/or physically. Our bodies know that it is good for us to cry after disaster and grief strike us. So, don't fight against our bodies' natural and normal processes; don't hold back tears."

"Interesting," the oncologist pondered. "So studies have actually shown that there are many physiological as well as emotional benefits to crying. I guess that's why kids automatically cry when they are in emotional distress."

"Yes," I replied. "Unfortunately, most adults feel that we should not cry because we subconsciously believe that if we do, then it means we are weak. Some of us even think that crying is something to be ashamed of. One reason for adults to believe that crying is shameful is that when we cry, people often leave us alone to 'give us space.' When they do this, it sends the message that we need to cry alone, implying that it is shameful to cry. Another reason adults often subconsciously believe it is inappropriate to cry is because when we cry as children, adults might tell us to 'stop crying,' or to 'go to your room' without explaining why. And lastly, many of us, as we grew up, were told to 'be strong, don't cry,' which implies that crying equates to being weak. Because of all these reasons, we as adults feel that crying is something to be ashamed of—a sign of weakness. The truth is, crying is a normal and natural process that our bodies do when we are in distress, and it is a sign of strength."

Crying is Being Strong

The oncologist now gave me a doubtful look. "How is crying a sign of strength? What about those cry-babies who cry from watching a movie?"

"Well, when we allow ourselves to cry after our hearts are broken, we are choosing to acknowledge and honor the grief so that we can fully move beyond it. Crying enables us to face our grief squarely, which can make us quite uncomfortable and vulnerable. Additionally, we must face every stigma about crying. It can be tempting to try to push the grief away when we are first struck by tragedy. However, our grief is like hot lava—we cannot push it away or run from it. We want to face it and allow it to flow away safely in order to heal from it completely. Still, it can be very uncomfortable to face our grief, and can leave us vulnerable to stigmas. To be willing to be uncomfortable in order to heal completely from our grief takes courage. It takes inner strength to be courageous," I said.

"And as for people who cry while watching a heartfelt movie or the news—they cry because their hearts have been touched by and opened with love. Just as our bodies know to release tears that help our emotional hearts heal when they have been broken open by the grief of our tragedies, our bodies release tears to nourish the seeds of love that people feel from viewing the movie or news. Still, it takes courage to be willing to be vulnerable and cry despite the stigma. So, crying is a sign of courage."

To my delight, the oncologist nodded. "So crying is good and crying is a sign of strength."

Dry Glue

"Yes," I replied. "And there is another reason why crying is very good for us when our hearts have been broken.

18

Have you ever tried washing dirty dishes with no water? What about trying to bond two things together with dry glue powder? Without water, we cannot wash our dirty dishes; without moisture, glue would not bind the pieces together. Our hearts have been broken into pieces by our grief, and our tears are the glue that we need to put them back together. Our tears are the water that allows us to wash away the 'dirt of life' that contaminates our hearts. So, not only is crying physiologically beneficial, but some crying is often necessary for us to clean up and put our broken hearts back together, even though it can be uncomfortable and make us feel vulnerable to cry.

"We can make our grief flow away with our tears. Just as the rain can reduce a wildfire, our tears can reduce the heat of the internal fire caused by our grief. Just as rainwater nourishes plants, our tears nourish our hearts. Just as the rain can wash away the ashes from a wildfire, our tears help to wash away the residue of our pain. Let our tears flow, and let our grief flow away with them. So, not only is it okay to cry when our hearts are broken, but it is *good* to cry, even if just for one minute. And yes, this applies to men too."

Several months after my conversation with the oncologist, she greeted me with a big smile. "I want to thank you again for talking to me about crying. When Dad was getting better, I told him about crying. Dad and I cry together now, when we are upset and when we are happy, and it has actually made us closer. Also, now I tell my patients that crying can be good. And they all say they feel better knowing that they can cry without thinking that it's weak and silly to cry."

MIDNIGHT THUMBS UP

"Daddy, please read me another bedtime story," I begged, not wanting to go to sleep yet.

Dad looked at me and smiled. "Okay, one more story." I was delightfully surprised, because he usually said no. Dad pulled out a thin book and started telling me a story about Ting-Ting the Magic Cat.

Ting-Ting had a big birthday party, and he got a lot of nice gifts. He got big parcels and small parcels, all nicely wrapped with colorful papers and bows, and Ting-Ting was very happy and excited to receive all these lovely gifts. At the end of the night, all the guests left, but Ting-Ting didn't want the party to stop. He wanted to keep enjoying nice gifts all year round, until his next birthday. So, Ting-Ting used his magic to make the gifts rewrap themselves at the end of the night, and he would open them again the next day. Every day for the whole year, Ting-Ting opened his lovely birthday gifts and had a lovely party, but when his birthday came around again, Ting-Ting was not happy.

"Why was he not happy, Daddy?" I asked.

"Because he had enjoyed his party all year round already, this time it wasn't special anymore. You see, even a nice party needs to stop. Even a fun party, if it doesn't stop, will not seem so nice anymore. All parties, fun or not, need to stop, so tomorrow you can have a different, even more delightful party."

I thought about it for a moment. "How do I know there will be a nicer party tomorrow, Daddy?"

Dad smiled again, "Because you believe, and you do what you need to do, like Cinderella. Cinderella's nice party had to stop, but she did not give up. She had her mouse friends help her so she could see the prince again after the first party was over, and then she became a princess. We need to stop reading stories now so tomorrow we can read a different, better bedtime story."

Don't Stay Over

Similar to how rain is needed to help plants grow, it is highly beneficial to cry when life throws rotten lemons at us. On the other hand, just as a full month of downpour will not be good for any plant, it is necessary for a pity party to eventually come to an end.

We want to acknowledge and honor our grief, but there is a huge difference between acknowledging the pain that we are feeling and allowing our tears to help us heal, versus dwelling on the pain. Just as we would not want to invite the police who came to us with a warrant to move in with us, we don't want to dwell on our pain. Dwelling on a broken heart is like rolling around in broken glass: it will create more pain, worsen the pain we already have, and keep us stuck in our misery.

We also don't want to rehash our interview with the police (or with our friends or foes) over and over in our mind for days and weeks to come. Replaying the event and stewing about the interview that is already in the past will only cause more anguish in us, while the police officers have long since left. Instead, we want to give the police interview the time it needs and then move on. We want to acknowledge, honor, and release our tears from our broken heart and release the event that caused our grief.

Was Cinderella Lucky?

Cinderella believed, and she took action with what she had. Even though she cried, Cinderella never gave up hope; she did what she had to do in order to survive through the dark chapters of her life. She believed that the sun would rise again and that her prince would come. She cast her eyes upon what she desired: a two-thumbs-up life as a princess. And with help from her friends, she made her dress, put it on, and went to the party.

Even though Cinderella cried after the party did not go as she had planned, she remained hopeful despite facing new obstacles. She kept believing in the possibility of a better future, and did what she could to improve her situation. She was sad but not bitter, and once an opportunity showed up, she took immediate action. She put her own foot into the magic glass slipper, believing still that the prince would realize that it was she who had worn the slipper the night before, and that he would continue to love the sweet girl that she was. It's a good thing that Cinderella did not become bitter, even with every travesty she experienced, for the prince might not have loved a bitter girl.

Choose "Two Thumbs Up" Now

We all have a Cinderella moment in our lives. Changes, both welcome and unwelcome, will happen in our lifetime. When a change brings us grief, we want to acknowledge it, honor it, and release our tears. Then, it is up to us to end the pity party and choose better over bitter. It is up to us to recognize that this is a dark chapter in our book of life, but we can choose for the next chapter to be one of recovery and possibility, as Mark did when his house was burned down by a wildfire. Only you can choose what to believe. If you do what it takes to survive the cold, dreary winter, you can have a two-thumbs-up spring. Only you can choose to take shelter during the storm, but you must remember to look up to see the rainbow once the storm calms down.

"How come you smile instead of whine and groan during the tough exercises?" my Pilates instructor curiously asked me after one particularly challenging advanced class.

"Because you amplify what you focus on, so I focus on the good," I said. The instructor looked confused, so I explained, "If you focus on the pain, you tend to feel more of the pain. If you focus on how good the exercise will make you feel and look afterward, you will feel less of the pain from the exercise even as you are doing it. If you smile, which releases feel-good endorphins and serotonin, you feel even less of your aching muscles as you go through the tough moves."

Focusing on the upcoming good instead of the pain

will help us better tolerate our pain. This technique works well when we are exercising our bodies. It also works well when we are going through life's tough exercises. Our challenging times are exercises and lessons from life, which help us to become even stronger. Now that you have decided to end your pity party and move on, move through your grief with a two-thumbs-up attitude toward the upcoming good, knowing full well that *every day, in every way, things are getting better and better.*

BEAUTIFULLY IMPERFECT

"Your feet and hips are not aligned perfectly," my Pilates instructor told me during an advanced class with complicated twisting and placement.

"Maybe it's just too advanced for me. Maybe I just can't do this," I replied with exasperation after trying to do the same exercise for four weeks in a row, each time discovering a new imperfection.

The instructor laughed, "No, it's not too advanced for you. And yes, you can do it. You did it fine last time when you stopped trying to think about it too much, when you stopped trying to do it perfectly."

I looked at her, confused and annoyed. "You just told me that I was not aligned perfectly, and now you say not to worry about doing things perfectly. Aren't we trying to have perfect alignments and movements?"

The instructor, who knows I am a recovering perfectionist, laughed again: "Trying. Trying is the key word. Try to do the best you can. Endeavor to do it better today than you did yesterday. Endeavor to be even better tomorrow than you are today. Nobody is perfect. Life is not perfect. No one makes a perfect move all the time, not even the advanced students and instructors. What's important is that you are getting better and better most of the time. Some days you tend to do worse than you did in the past, maybe because you are having a bad day; that's okay. We know that nothing is perfect; no one makes perfect moves all the time."

When we start a new exercise, we often do the moves imperfectly. Even the advanced students and instructors make imperfect moves. We are all students of life, and we all make mistakes. As we navigate through our emotional disasters, imperfect moves are inevitable. We have some great days, but there will be days when we can barely look at our thumbs, much less have a two-thumbs-up attitude. This is fine. Even a robot needs maintenance at times. We are human. We are meant to have good days, great days, and not so good days. We are meant to be imperfect. Perfection is not the goal. Perfection in doing the steps, and in remembering the details discussed in this book, should never be our goal—because perfection is not important. What's important is doing the best that we can by taking one step at a time in order to have a two-thumbs-up attitude, knowing and believing that *every day, in every way, things are getting better and better.*

REVIEW

1. Acknowledge and honor our feelings and grief.
2. Grief is like an invisible abscess.
3. Grief is cumulative, and cumulatively destructive.[1]
4. Let go of resistance.
5. Crying is good.
6. Do not dwell.
7. Have a two-thumbs-up attitude now.
8. This is a dark chapter, but you can choose not to let it be the rest of your book of life.
9. Nothing is perfect.

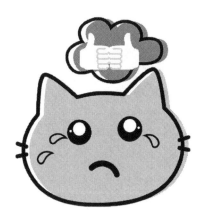

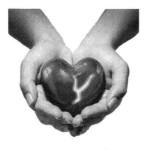

Chapter 2

CHAMELEON FINGERPRINT

The second step for navigating through our disaster comes from our second finger, the pointer finger. Just as it helps us to have some clear understanding of math when we do algebra, it's helpful to have an understanding of grief when navigating through the dark valleys of our lives. In this chapter, we are going to "index" grief so that we can understand it better, even when it takes us by surprise. This way, we will be able to know which direction to point toward so that we can move with more ease as we navigate through the dark valley of our lives.

CHAMELEON

Grief is like a chameleon. Even when there is death or divorce, the grief associated with it might not present itself as sadness. When the cause of our grief is something other than an apparent loss, it is even more likely that the grief will present itself as anything but sadness. Knowing about this "chameleon" is very important for us to be able to recognize that we are grieving, and thus address the underlying feelings appropriately.

Loveless Honeymoon

"Sorry I am so late. I forgot what day it was," my friend Rina apologized as she dashed into the oceanfront café where I had been waiting for her.

"Don't worry; I'm not in a rush. It's so great to see you again, Rina. You look great! How are you? How was your private African safari trip?" I greeted my friend.

"I'm well. So great to be at the beach again. The trip was okay. It was for our belated honeymoon," Rina said flatly.

I intuitively sensed a problem: "How's married life?"

"Married life's okay," she said with a forced smile. "You know, I prefer big cities, like Los Angeles, and I prefer to be close to the beach."

I pondered, "Oh! I thought San Diego was a big city too, and your home is on a semi-private beach there. How's your husband, Ray?"

"He's fine; his work is good." She stared quietly at the ocean for a couple of minutes and then said, "Lately,

28

Ray has just been irritating me. He says I have become a workaholic and act like the Energizer Bunny on steroids. I think he's just too slow and unmotivated."

"Oh! Wow! You used to call him Mr. Super-Achiever, with his quick mind and great successes," I blurted out before I could stop myself.

Rina looked irritated: "He still is, but he doesn't like me working ten to twelve hours a day, seven days a week, even though I work from home. He says I'm too high strung, too easily agitated, and cold now."

"Cold? Like physically cold?" I asked.

Rina blew a sharp exhale. "No. Well, yes, that too. But more like emotionless. I just don't feel close to him anymore."

My intuition was right; Rina was having a problem. "I see. You are one of the sweetest, warmest, calmest people I know, and a master at work-life balance. Are you working the whole week because your business is in trouble?" I asked her, to clarify where her trouble was.

"My business is still doing great. Strangely, it's not growing much at all, even with me working an extra 30 to 40 percent more a week. I'm just not able to focus well lately. No, I'm not working like a slave because I need to; I just don't have many things to do down in San Diego. All my friends and family are here, and Ray is busy at work. I don't know the area or the neighbors. I don't think my super-affluent, snooty neighbors even like me. I don't feel like I fit in. I feel a little like Cinderella, alone and lost in the palace, so I just work more."

I let Rina get lost in her thoughts for a moment and then asked her, "Is it possible that you work more and subconsciously try to numb yourself so you don't feel as much of your pain from the sudden changes? Perhaps you might be agitated and hyperactive because you feel lost? Over time, maybe those feelings got worse from the new tension with your husband and overworking yourself?"

Rina thought about it for a moment, then her shoulders lowered. "I think you're right," she said, as tears started to fill her eyes.

Who would think that marrying one's prince charming could bring with it so much emotional turmoil? We know that we are supposed to be happy when we get married, and we really are happy when it happens. However, along with the marriage come changes, particularly if we have to move. When we must relocate for our marriage, we may experience emotional turmoil from the drastic lifestyle change. Another name for emotional turmoil is grief.

Unfortunately, most people think that grief only comes with death, divorce, or a dire medical diagnosis. Most people don't know that grief is "the conflicting feelings caused by a change in our familiar routine," and that there are over forty causes of grief.[1] This simply means that any change that can cause us to experience stress or emotional turmoil may cause grief as well. In other words, having a new family member, moving, experiencing an illness or an accident, getting a new job, going to college, witnessing a horrific event, getting married, and many other events that bring a change in our familiar routine can cause grief.

One reason it can be difficult for us to recognize that we are grieving is that grief is a great chameleon. Often it does not come knocking on our door as sadness. Have you ever seen a lava lamp? Grief is like the lava that can change its look and color. It sneaks and seeps into your life in many different forms and emotions. Not realizing that they might be grieving makes it challenging for most people to realize what they are actually going through. Being unaware of our grief is quite unfortunate because we will not be able to heal from our emotional trauma appropriately.

In Rina's case, her grief disguised itself as forgetfulness, agitation, inability to focus, overactivity, emotionlessness, and irritability. Looking back, Rina recalled feeling deep sadness with her move and marriage. She felt sadness from having to leave what she grew up with, the freedom of living alone, her supportive friends, and even the Los Angeles traffic jams she had learned to navigate and outsmart. However, believing that she should feel only happiness, Rina immediately tried to push away her sadness instead of addressing it.

Unfortunately, unresolved grief often causes subconscious resentment toward what or whom we perceive as the cause of the grief. In the case of a marriage, our unresolved grief can subconsciously lead us to resent our new spouse. This resentment toward our spouse makes us unable to form connections, and we lose our emotional closeness as a result. It is very normal to feel conflicting emotions when we get married. We want to address the sadness appropriately in order to avoid starting our marriage with unresolved grief and to prevent more problems in the future. Thankfully for Rina, she allowed me to help her take the necessary steps to resolve her wedding grief. Rina is now in a much better relationship with her husband. Since she is back to her sweet, warm, cheerful self, her previously "snooty" neighbors are friendly toward her too. Rina is now thriving in her new palace and her new neighborhood.

The Retirement Trap

"My husband and I are thinking about getting a divorce after thirty-eight years of marriage," Nancy, my prospective client, told me.

"Oh dear! Can you tell me more, please?" I asked her.

Tears started to pool in Nancy's eyes. "Well, my husband retired two years ago, and we just can't stand each other now, so we are getting a divorce."

"I'm sorry to hear that. Looking back, how was your relationship before the retirement?" I asked.

Nancy didn't even have to think about it, "It was great. That's the sad thing. We had a great relationship, and both of us were looking forward to his retirement. There were things he always wanted to do, places we planned on visiting. And I was looking forward to having him at home during the day after having the house all to myself all these years."

"I see. What's been going on since your husband's retirement? Is he doing the things he wanted to do?" I asked.

Nancy shook her head, "No, not all. He doesn't do any of them. All my husband does now is sleep during the day because he doesn't sleep well at night. He gets in my way and complains a lot. He's become so negative and lazy. Lately, he rarely plays golf or goes hiking with me the way he used to on the weekends. We were supposed to visit my sister for a week last month, but he didn't even want to go. We ended up only going for three days because all he did was sleep and complain. He should be happy that he's retired, but I think it's only made him depressed."

"Has he been seen by a doctor? How's his health?" I inquired.

"His health is fine," Nancy informed me. "He had a full checkup and a clean bill of health just a couple of months ago. I guess I just never knew him well when he was working because he wasn't with me all the time. Now that he is around all day, I get to see his true colors. I'm stressed out and confused, and it's giving me panic attacks."

I explained to Nancy that both she and her husband might be grieving. Retirement is a common cause of grief, of which many people are unaware. Just as when we get married or when our child has left home to go to college, retiring causes an abrupt change in our routine. This significant change in the routine of everyone involved can cause grief. When we are grieving, we often behave and think differently than usual. Unaware of their grief, each grief-stricken family member often creates conflict among themselves. These conflicts add even more to the antagonistic feelings that arise from the changes in our routine. Unrecognized and unresolved, this whole process becomes a circle of destruction, many times leading to animosity and even divorce.

Another reason for a retiree to experience grief is that many people identify themselves with what they do, and retirement can make them feel as if they have lost their identity.

Nancy's husband's apathy, isolation, depression, abnormal sleeping pattern, irritability, anger, and negativity, as well as Nancy's panic attacks and numbness, are all common disguises of grief.

Nancy thought for a moment. "Even if he is grieving, my husband would never believe it. There's no way he would even listen to me now since we basically yell at each other every time we talk these days. That's why we are getting a divorce; we are just not on the same page anymore."

"Well, since you are grieving from not being on the same page anymore with your husband, how about if we take care of you for now and see how things are after six to eight weeks?" I suggested. "Put on your own oxygen mask first. You will learn the basic tools and skills that could be beneficial in navigating and recovering from your grief with more ease. It will help you immediately, and if you do end up going through a divorce, the lifelong skills and tools you have gained from the coaching will be useful to help you again." Nancy decided to allow me to help her work on her grief and her feelings.

After Nancy completed her last class, she came to me and said: "Thank you—I don't think we are getting a divorce anymore. My husband has stopped snapping at me for at least a few weeks now. Last night, he thanked me for making dinner and for being so patient with his grumbling. He used to thank me for making dinner, but not since he retired. I know I have not been resenting him or yelling at him with all the progress we made." Her cell phone signaled a text from her husband. She read the text and looked up with a big grin. "My husband wants to work with you. When can he start?"

Nancy's husband started that week. At his last class, he told me that his relationship with Nancy was the best it had been since his retirement. "Would you like anything from Siberia? Nancy and I are going for two weeks on a trans-Siberian train trip. That's the first item on our Trip Bucket List," he said with a big, happy grin.

Explosive Edith

"How could you be so immoral, stealing another woman's husband and ruining their family?" Edith, my usually gentle and soft-spoken best friend, yelled at my cousin as the three of us stood in a Starbucks line. My cousin's face showed surprise, confusion, and then irritation. I looked at Edith with a puzzled expression, unable to figure out where her comment had came from, since my cousin had said nothing about being involved with anyone and I knew that she was not stealing anyone's husband.

"Ummm, what made you say that, Edith?" I tried to ask gently, but Edith snapped at me in return.

"You don't think it's immoral to be sleeping with a married man?" Edith asked. "Can you imagine how the wife must feel? And the poor kids? It will traumatize them for the rest of their lives! If you don't think it's immoral, then there's something wrong with you too!"

"I'm sorry, I did not ask my question clearly," I said, diplomatically. "What made you think that my cousin is sleeping with a married man?"

Edith pointed at my cousin and snapped back, "That's what she just implied, you didn't catch that? Actually, I'm done shopping. I have to go home," and she stomped away.

We all went home because now my cousin was annoyed, and I felt disturbed by the whole incident.

Later that week, I found out that Edith's father had had a mistress when she was growing up. During those years, he would frequently miss important dates for Edith, such as school events and even her eleventh birthday. This created a lot of disappointment and resentment in Edith. After a few years, Edith's father returned to his family and soon everyone acted as if nothing had ever happened. This forced Edith to bury the feelings of betrayal she had toward her father, and the pain never went away as a result.

The only problem with trying to bury grief, whether

the disaster is emotional, physical, or both, is that grief behaves like hot lava. Just as hot lava inside of a mountain builds pressure from the physical heat, the emotional heat from unresolved grief often manifests as anger and builds pressure inside of us. We might misinterpret what others say and get very angry at them for something they didn't do or say. Irritability, lingering anger, and overreacting (or "exploding") inappropriately, as well as hypersensitivity to a subject, are common manifestations of unresolved grief. If left unresolved, this will only get worse. Just like hot lava, grief is cumulative and cumulatively destructive,[1] burning us from the inside. Instead of burying it, we want to recognize and resolve it.

Eighteen Scars of Shame

"So, how come you don't have any kids?" Anya, my long-lost college friend, asked me.

"Well, I guess I've never felt strongly called to having my own kids," I said.

"Oh! I see. Actually, I didn't think you even liked kids that much, at least not when we were in college," she said.

Her comment made me think about something: "What about you? I remember that you loved kids. Why don't you have any?"

Anya didn't answer my question, but instead she changed the subject. "So, what's the wildest thing you have seen grievers do?" she asked me.

"The wildest thing? What do you mean?" I asked to clarify.

37

"You know, like they kill someone or burn their own home or hurt themselves because of their grief," she said impatiently.

I thought about it. "I don't personally know of anyone killing anyone else or burning their own home. Sadly, I have seen people hurt themselves from grief."

"So, you know some crazies?" Anya inquired.

"I don't think they are crazy; what they need is love and help in order to heal their emotional pain. I think it is very sad to be in such deep emotional pain, and often emotional isolation, that they resort to hurting themselves. My heart goes out to those in such pain," I replied, curious about the direction of the conversation.

"You don't think this is crazy?" Anya pulled up one side of her blouse to show a long scab, a couple of scars, and several tattoo lines on her waist. I surely didn't expect to see this.

"What caused these cuts?" I asked.

"Every cut is a year that she would have lived if I had not aborted her instead," Anya said with chilling calmness. "I got nine on the other waist. This one was from last week, which would have been her eighteenth birthday. If the cut didn't make a scar, I put a tattoo after the wound healed to remind me of the monster I am and the punishment I deserve. I'm not grieving. I am guilty of a shameful sin, and I don't deserve ever to have a child again. So, do you still believe I'm not crazy? By the way, no one else knows about this, not even my mother, so if this gets back to me, I'll know you spilled my secret," Anya looked at me intensely.

"Anya, you are not crazy, and I promise I will not tell anyone about this," I replied. "Crazy is a very loose term. Google's online dictionary defines crazy as 'mentally deranged.' You are cutting yourself because you are feeling so much pain from what you believe is a shameful sin. But sin is a very relative term. What is a sin for one person can be a virtue for another. I am not going to say anything definitive about abortion, but I suspect you had yours because you believed, at least eighteen years ago, that it was the best option for her and you and everyone involved."

Anya's eyes started to water as she nodded quietly, then started sobbing uncontrollably as she drew her knees up to her chest on the chair.

"Oh, Anya. My heart goes out to you. I can only imagine how you have felt for so long with all this shame and guilt you have. I can only imagine the depth of the pain you are experiencing. You might think you are not grieving, but shame and guilt can cause us to grieve intensely. You, and most people who hurt themselves because of grief, typically do it because they feel lost and are in deep pain. Prolonged guilt and shame very often cause deep, isolating emotional pain. Sadly, shame is what makes many of these grievers the last to reach out for help. You are not crazy, and you do not need to be punished. What you need is help with your shame, guilt, and grief so you can have peace of mind again."

Thankfully, Anya allowed me to help her release her guilt and shame, and recover from her grief.

Three years had passed since I discovered Anya's shame and guilt when I received a text from her saying, "Would you like to be a godmother to my soon-to-be-here daughter?"

I texted back "I'd LOVE to!" and then called her. Anya told me that shortly after she completed her Moving Beyond Grief work with me, she met a wonderful gentleman.

"I told him about the abortion* and the cutting I did for eighteen years. And to my surprise, he thanked me for trusting him and for being vulnerable with him. He told me he loved and respected me just as much. I am so grateful to have people like you and him and my mom and sister—who I also told about my secret—who love and accept me as I am," Anya said.

"I am very happy for you, Anya. Congratulations," I told her.

"Thank you. Yes, I am very happy. The baby actually brought my fiancé and me closer together, too. We are going to get married, and have the baptism in the summer, and we both want you to be my maid of honor and her godmother. If it wasn't for your help, I still wouldn't even be dating again."

Anya and her husband had a very beautiful wedding and baptism, and I am very grateful and honored to have been able to help her recover from her grief and thrive again.

---

* The author does not approve or disapprove abortion or any religious belief or practice. Anya (name has been changed), upon recovering from her grief fully, has allowed the author to share her story whenever appropriate, to be able to help others.

The Yogis and Einstein

"Hi! It's been a few years since I saw you. How are you?" my wise old acupuncturist greeted me enthusiastically.

"Oh! My neck and hip pain resolved on their own. I am here because my back has been hurting for a few weeks now; I might have pulled it," I replied.

"Oh wow! Your neck and hip pain resolved completely? When did that happen? And what did you do for it?" She appeared so curious, since I previously had chronic neck and hip pain that was not responsive to any medical treatment from any doctor or chiropractor.

"I noticed both the neck and hip pain were gone almost two years ago," I said. "I didn't do anything differently. I stopped coming because I went through a divorce, even though you were outstanding in keeping me comfortable."

My acupuncturist nodded her head, "When was your divorce? How was your marriage, truthfully, before the divorce?"

With my new knowledge about grief, emotions, and energy, I knew why the wise acupuncturist asked that. I smiled at her, "The divorce was finalized a little over two years ago, a few months before I noticed that my neck and hip pain went away out of the blue. The marriage, well, let's just say it was not as perfect as I wanted it to be."

She nodded as if she knew already. "Yes. So not only did you have a pain-in-the-neck marriage, you were trying to deny it and suppress your feelings. You know, the yogis say that we hold our feelings in our hips. Remember

41

you used to say you wanted to cry when I helped you stretch your hip? That's because you were holding your grief there. Well, let's look at your back now." The wise acupuncturist worked on my back, and I felt less pain by the end of the session.

"Come back in one week," she said. She paused, pointed to my heart, and continued, "During the week, see what's holding you back." I knew the answer the moment she said it—this time I chose to be honest with myself and take actions to resolve the circumstances. My back pain went away without the second visit and never recurred.

Albert Einstein said, "Everything is energy, and that's all there is to it." This means that our emotions are energy, and so is our physical body. Since both are energy, it makes perfect sense that a disturbance in one will have an impact on the other. Our emotional and physical states affect each other. Just as a significant or prolonged physical illness often causes us to grieve, it is common for us to experience physical symptoms in addition to emotional symptoms when an emotional disaster affects us. Physical symptoms such as shortness of breath, irregular menstruation, oversensitivity to noise and light, dry mouth, and others can all be a physical disguise of grief. Unresolved grief may also manifest physically as chronic, inexplicable aches and pains, digestive problems, persistent fatigue, and even actual physical illness.

The Shape-Shifting Chameleon

Grief is like a shape-shifting chameleon. Depending on

who you are and what causes your grief, you might not feel any sadness at all. Rather than sadness, many people can feel irrationally angry toward someone or something else. In fact, in my work as an oncologist, many family members of the deceased patients have expressed a lot more anger or guilt than sadness. They are angry at the doctors, at themselves, and at life. Often, this anger is exacerbated by guilt from believing that they should have done things differently, while the truth is that they did the best they could with the information, resources, and awareness that they had.

Anger is one of the most common disguises of grief. We become angry because we feel powerless for not being able to change the tragedy. We might also become angry if we think that we have been treated unfairly. Fear is also a very common cause of anger. When a tragedy strikes us, we might be fearful of not knowing how tomorrow is going to be, and in turn, we feel powerless and angry. Additionally, we feel vulnerable when our hearts are broken. This vulnerability is normal and natural, but it often makes us feel very uncomfortable, and this discomfort can lead to anger.

Another common disguise of grief is depression. Depression can cause grief, and emotional pain can cause depression. Other common disguises of grief are forgetfulness, agitation, inability to focus, overactivity, irritability, apathy, negativity, panic attacks, emotional numbness, insomnia, and the physical symptoms discussed previously. Knowing grief and its many disguises is very beneficial, as it allows us to recognize when we or someone we care about is grieving, and thus be able to address it promptly.

FINGERPRINT

Grief is like our fingerprints. Have you ever looked closely at your fingerprints? Notice that each of your fingers has a similar, but not identical, pattern to the others. Grief is like our fingerprints in that no two people feel the exact same grief, even if they have grown up together and are observing the same tragedy at same time. Similarly, the same person experiencing two very similar events, such as the death of a beloved pet, might feel differently each time. For this reason, there is no right or wrong way for any of us to grieve.

Lost on the Stage

"Sorry I'm late. I backed up into my own fence just now like an idiot," said Nadia, the new client whose husband had died in his sleep, as she rushed into my office. I let her have a seat before I let her know that her appointment was for the next day.

When I told her, Nadia buried her face in her hands. "Okay, I am going crazy. Stupid me, I should have double-checked my calendar before coming today, knowing how scatterbrained I am lately. Silly me, backed up into my own fence just now when I should have driven forward. I am just a lost cause, so much so that I can't even fit in those grief stages. I'm just a crazy, stupid weirdo." Her tears started to well up.

"The grief stages?" I asked, "Do you mean the Five Stages of Grief popularized by Dr. Elizabeth Kubler-Ross?"

Nadia nodded. "Yes, that. I have been so sad and depressed ever since my husband died. I feel worse every day. My friend who studied psychology told me that it is because I skipped the other three stages. I didn't have denial, because what's to deny? Paul is gone, peacefully in his sleep, and I'm not angry about it. My friend told me that I need to be angry in order to feel better. I am sad that he is gone, but it was exactly the way he wanted it, healthy and living life well until the end. He went to sleep and never woke up again. My friend said that I should be angry at him for leaving me. That sounds so crazy to me. He was twenty-five years older than I am; I knew he would leave before I do, and he lived until ninety. I didn't even expect to have forty years with him, so I'm grateful for it. At the same time, I feel so depressed, and I feel stupid because I can't shake it off or get angry. My friend said that I accepted his passing too quickly and that's why I am depressed."

I explained to Nadia that the "five stages of grief" concept (denial, anger, bargaining, depression, and acceptance) was designed only for people facing a terminal illness. It was not designed to explain grief from other causes.[1] Even people who experience terminal illness do not always follow the stages in an orderly manner or the timeline for each stage. Some people with a terminal illness go through each of the stages very quickly, but do not stay in acceptance. They experience temporary acceptance, but then go backward, start over, jump around, or cycle through the stages. Unfortunately, many people are not aware of the fact that the five stages of grief were created specifically for people with a terminal illness—this is one of the most common misunderstandings in navigating grief.

Many of us believe that when we are grieving, we need to follow the five stages of grief step-by-step in a certain timeframe. When we don't do so, we feel that there is something wrong with us. Then we feel bad not only from our grief but also from a misunderstanding about grief, when in fact, everyone grieves differently each time. Grief and feelings do not follow an exact order and timeline. Our grieving is like our fingerprints. Just as there is no good or bad, right or wrong, normal or abnormal fingerprint, there are no good or bad, right or wrong, normal or abnormal feelings and ways of grieving. We are all individuals, and we should expect to feel in our own personal way when changes happen in our lives. Also, we can never really know how we will feel about any event until a change occurs, just as we can never really know how someone else feels about something either.

No Resuscitation

Pauline, my emergency veterinarian friend, texted me, "Do you want to go get some wine, like now? I'll treat."

She knows I don't drink wine unless I'm at a party, and I know that's her way of saying she needs to vent to me. I told her that she could just come over to my home, and she arrived in ten minutes, looking annoyed.

"What happened?" I asked.

"It's a crazy busy day with even crazier people, complete insanity," Pauline answered.

"Please tell me more," I said.

Pauline proceeded to vent about having two staff members call in sick, etc., etc., and, "Oh! As if that wasn't enough, the last clients were a total disaster. They came in with a drowned old blind dog. I successfully resuscitated the dog, but when I told them the great news they screamed at me. They told me that I'm unethical and they didn't want to pay." Pauline's face turned red as she fumed.

"I'm so sorry to hear that," I said.

"Yeah, they told me that I should have let the dog die since he was old, senile, blind, and he belonged to their very handicapped mother who's moving into a nursing home. The dog won't be able to go to the nursing home with the mom and wouldn't do well with their two young kids. I didn't know, and they signed the CPR order. How could I know that they'd be happier if the dog stayed dead?"

I assured Pauline that she could not have known, since we can never really know how someone else might feel over a loss. In fact, many people who are prolonged caretakers for loved ones with a terminal condition feel more relief than sadness when the person they have been caring for dies. This is not selfish; this is just normal. Caretakers often go through anticipatory grief: the grief of the looming loss. In addition, they often experience the grief of being in an unpleasant situation. For these reasons, many caretakers feel a sense of relief when the person they are taking care of dies. This is very normal, for it is in our nature to want to be able to heal our hearts and move on.

Roscoe

June 20, 2013. The chatty old lady neighbor saw me standing on my patio and invited herself to stop by. "Where's your old grey cat? I usually see him at the window but not the last week or so." I had not known that she and the cat had been watching each other all the while.

"He passed away," I said. "He suddenly got sick and died five days later."

She looked at me kindly. "Oh no! I'm so sorry. He was a good-looking cat, seemed nice too. How old was he?"

I took a deep breath; I did not feel like chatting about my cat. "He was twenty."

"Wow! That's really good, most cats die long before that."

I thought to myself, "So? He's not most cats. He's not at all like the other cats I've had."

The old lady continued yapping, "I know it's still

tough. I lost my old cat a couple of years ago too. I know exactly how you feel."

Really? I'm sure that she and her seven cats don't know exactly how I feel. Roscoe was not just a cat. He was my best friend, my boy, my guardian angel. He was by my side when I was studying, when I was sick, when my former husband left.

The old neighbor continued, "Well, at least you still have another cat. Don't you have another one? I'll help you get another cat too. I know how it is."

But she didn't know how it was for me. She didn't even know that Roscoe was my only friend, the only one I could fully trust, and the only one who accepted me as I was. She had no idea. Not to mention that the other cat, my last cat, followed Roscoe and died nine days after him. No one knew how painful it had been for me to suffer one tragedy after another for two years straight. In my mind, no one could possibly even start to imagine how I felt.

We can never know exactly how someone feels at any given point in time, whether it is a joyful event or a tragic one. Now that we know this, we should also know not to say "I know how you feel," even if we have had a similar loss.

Heart with Ears on Open Hands (GRM)

Instead of telling a grieving person that we know how they feel or forcing ourselves to feel emotions that come to us naturally, let's just be a heart with ears and open hands.

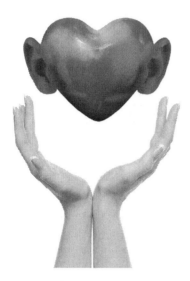

Let's be a heart with ears: listen with compassion and no judgment.[1]

Let's truly listen with love and patience to ourselves and others during tough times. Too often, we judge ourselves harshly when we do things that we wish we had not done or said in the past. What we want to remember is that, when we are having a tough time, we have been thrown off our normal state of mind. Too often, we tell ourselves that we are silly/stupid/crazy/weird because we don't do what we ourselves, or others, expect us to do.

It is very normal for us to talk harshly to ourselves when we feel that we are not doing our best, because it is in our human nature to desire to do the best that we can. Instead of being harsh, let's be kind and patient with ourselves. Let's be a heart with ears for ourselves. Let's listen with compassion and without judgment when we notice that we are talking harshly to ourselves. We want to be kind and patient with ourselves when we notice that we are not doing what we think we should do, say, or think.

In addition to being a "heart with ears" to ourselves, we also want to have open hands when we are going through a tough time. Just as Cinderella allowed her mouse friends to help her survive through her tough time, we want to allow ourselves to receive support when we need it most. We want to have open hands, not gripping hands or tight fists. We want to be able to receive support, but not expect it to happen exactly the way we think it should. We want to be able to receive support as long as it is offered, but not become dependent upon it. For our own personal betterment, let's be a heart with ears and have open hands for support.

Let's also be a heart with ears and have open hands for others who are grieving. Let's listen to them with love and kindness. People want to be heard, and grievers need to be heard. They need to be able to safely share their feelings without being told what to do or how to feel. When we tell someone what to do/think/feel, we imply that we do not accept them or their thoughts and feelings. When we tell grievers what to do/think/feel, they might get the impression that we think they are doing something wrong.

Grievers often already feel like there's something wrong with them, and they are typically very sensitive to feeling unaccepted. The best thing for us to do is to listen without trying to give advice. Just listen with love and kindness and open hands. Offer them your support but do not impose it or expect them to receive it. Since we do not know how anyone else might feel, we don't want to say, "I know how you feel." We can instead say, "I am sorry. I am here for you. Let me know if I can help in any way."

REVIEW

1. Grief is not only from death or divorce. Grief is the conflicting feelings caused by a change in our familiar routine.
2. There are over forty causes of grief, including "supposed to be happy" events.
3. Grief is like a chameleon. It often disguises itself as many emotional and physical symptoms.
4. Guilt and shame can cause intense, isolating grief.
5. Grief is like our fingerprint. There is no right or wrong way to grieve.
6. "The Five Stages of Grief" developed by Dr. Kubler-Ross (denial, anger, bargaining, depression, and acceptance) were designed only for people facing a terminal illness.
7. We don't know how other people really feel.
8. Be a heart with ears and open hands, for ourselves and for others.

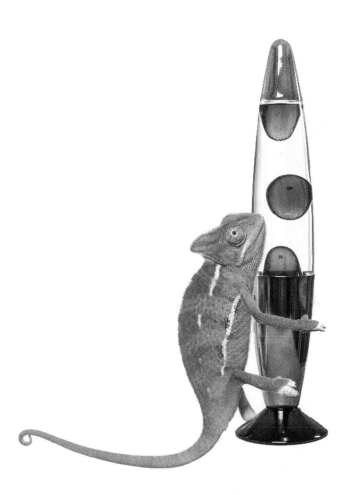

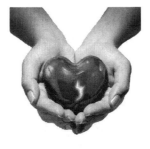

Chapter 3

MUDDLED IN THE MIDDLE

The third step for navigating through our disaster and the grief associated with it comes from our third finger: our middle finger. In western culture, starting as far back as the early Greek and Roman civilizations, we have raised our middle finger when we want to insult someone. We also raise our middle finger when someone offends us and we want to respond in kind. There are speculations, but no one knows for certain what triggered humans to start this response that originated in ancient times and transferred into our modern society. Perhaps the answer lies in our energy system. In the traditional Chinese medicine system, the middle finger represents the heart. The point for "heart" in Chinese acupressure system is in the middle of our middle finger.[5] Perhaps we instinctively raise our middle finger when we feel our heart has been violated and we want to stand up for ourselves. When we feel that our heart has been "stepped on," perhaps we instinctively hold up our middle finger to stand our ground. In this chapter, we will discuss various ways to understand and heal our hearts, no matter what damage was done. We do this by un-muddling our misunderstandings about grief, and healing our hearts with love and understanding.

UN-MUDDLING THE MISUNDERSTANDING

Grief is not a fun subject. Schools don't teach about grief, and thus we grow up having little understanding of it. The few little tidbits we learn about navigating our broken hearts after emotional disaster often come from friends and family, most of whom have no education or training about grief. No surprise, there is a widespread misunderstanding about grief and healing a broken heart. In this section, we will un-muddle this misunderstanding so that we can heal our broken hearts smoothly.

NOT a Broken Loser

"I do want to warn you that I am a flaw, an ungrateful, complete loser," Fawn, the new client, told me as she signed our agreement to work together.

"Oh! Thank you for the warning. Please tell me more," I replied without telling her that, unfortunately, many of my clients have felt the same way prior to us working together. Fawn proceeded to tell me that immediately after she had a miscarriage over one year ago, her friends were very supportive to her. For the first few months after the loss of her unborn son, her friends accompanied her constantly, kept her busy, took her to parties, and even sent her on a vacation.

"I felt less sad during the vacation and at the parties, but when I got home, I was just as sad," she told me. "I cried every time I saw the guest bedroom that would have become the baby's bedroom. After six months or so, my friends told me that it was time to move on. They took me on vacation again, but this time I didn't feel any better. I was still sad during the last vacation, and I am tired of the parties now. Every time I go to a party, I come back exhausted and sadder. I am exhausted from trying to put on a brave smiling face. I moved too, staying at my friend's duplex, so I would no longer see the baby's future bedroom. But I don't feel any better. Instead, I start to feel like I'm running from myself, and I feel suffocated at the new home. My friends tell me that I should be grateful that I still have twin daughters, but hearing them say that just makes me want to vomit. I am grateful for my twins, and I love them very much, but now every time I see them I feel more and more pain in my heart. I feel like I am almost resenting them now, which makes me feel even guiltier."

Fawn started to cry. "I'm such a bad mom, I couldn't keep the baby in my belly alive and now I feel like I'm also losing my twins. I'm such a miserable, ungrateful loser. I keep thinking maybe I did something wrong that made me lose my baby, maybe I was guilty of something in the past and this is the punishment, and I wonder why I can't just move on after all this time. All my friends tell me that I should have moved on by now, but I can't. I don't really want to because I love my baby even though he was never born. I don't want to move on and forget him." She pointed to her head and continued, "I think I am just sick, you know, mentally ill, to be in more pain now when I should feel much better. I guess I'm just a broken, ungrateful loser. That's why I'm here, but I don't know if you want to deal with a broken, ungrateful loser like me."

I handed her the tissue box. "You are not a loser, and you are not broken. You have a broken heart that has not been healed properly. Just like an abscess that is not properly treated, your yet-to-be-treated broken heart makes you feel worse over time. Unfortunately, there is a lot of misunderstanding about heartbreak and grief in our society. Even more unfortunately, our well-meaning friends and loved ones give us advice from this muddled information that makes us feel even worse, trapped and suffocating in the middle of the quicksand that is grief. What we want to do is to clarify this misunderstanding, which will effectively help you to heal perfectly well, stop feeling guilty, and stop feeling like a 'broken loser.'"

You are Whole and Courageous.

Would you consider yourself a "broken loser" if you had an infected broken leg caused by an earthquake that knocked you off your feet? Imagine that your infected broken leg received inappropriate medical treatment from well-intending friends who were not medical doctors, and the infection and the break got worse over time. Would you consider yourself a broken loser then? Most people would say that they had very bad luck, not that they were a broken loser.

It is the same when we have broken hearts. When disasters happen to us and leave us with broken hearts, we are not "losers" or "broken people."[1] We are whole and wonderful. You might feel that you cannot go on anymore, but this does not mean that you are a "loser" or a "broken person." Unfortunately, widespread misunderstanding about grief and broken hearts causes many people to think that they are broken when it is only their heart that is broken. You are whole and courageous, even though you have a broken heart that needs to heal completely using proper information, skills, and love. It takes courage to acknowledge what you have been through. It also takes courage for you to want to be able to learn and heal. Kudos to you for your courage and willingness to do what it takes to thrive again. You are a wonderful and courageous person.

Time Does NOT Heal All

Another common misunderstanding about grief is that time alone will heal your broken heart.[1] Imagine that you have a bleeding and infected broken leg. It won't do us any good to just sit with it in our living room, hoping it will fix itself. A broken leg will not heal itself well, even if the broken pieces eventually reunite. Without treatment, the infection in the broken leg will get worse and spread. With an infected broken leg, we need to acknowledge it and have it treated by appropriate physicians to resolve the infection and properly repair the break.

When a disaster strikes us, it leaves us with a broken heart. The grief that comes from our disaster is like an insidious infection of our mind and spirit. Untreated grief causes problems such as post-traumatic stress disorder, chronic depression, panic attacks, and physical symptoms, in addition to impairing our judgment and robbing us of our peace of mind and joy.[1] Time alone will not heal our broken hearts completely and smoothly. Just as we want to receive treatment from the appropriate physicians for our infected broken leg, we also want to receive guidance from compassionate, skillful, and knowledgeable experts in grief resolution in order to help us heal our broken hearts and clear out our grief.

Staying Busy Does Not Allow Healing.

Imagine you have a broken leg and you continue to keep walking on it for weeks. Not only will the walking not allow the leg to heal, but soon the broken pieces will become worse and more difficult to repair. This is the same as when we keep ourselves busy when we have a broken heart.

Keeping ourselves busy when we have a broken heart does not allow our hearts to heal.[1] At first, we might feel better when we are busy because our bodies release our natural epinephrine (adrenalin) to keep us going when we are wounded. As time goes by, the pain from our still-bleeding, broken hearts becomes stronger—so strong that distraction cannot keep our minds off our pain. This is the reason why Fawn did not feel better during her "second vacation that was meant to help her feel better." Her emotional pain was so severe that even distraction could not take her mind off it anymore. As time goes by, we exhaust our body's natural adrenalin that has been helping us feel much better while we are busy. We become exhausted when we force ourselves to be on the move. This is why Fawn found the parties exhausting and no longer fun.

Distraction, whether through parties, alcohol, sex, food, shopping, etc., works very temporarily. Distraction is like putting a bandage on the profusely gushing wound on your broken leg. A bandage can temporarily cover the wound, but it will not stop the bleeding. Even worse, over time, the bandage itself will cause a secondary problem of skin irritation. The parties, alcohol, and shopping can cause secondary problems in our lives, all while our broken hearts continue to bleed and our pain worsens. Distracting ourselves to avoid feeling the pain from our broken hearts or forcing ourselves to keep going does not allow our broken hearts to heal. Instead, it potentially makes it more difficult to heal. Just as when we have a broken leg, we want to rest and take the time we need to heal our hearts.

Running or Hiding is Futile

Fawn said, "I start to feel like I'm running from myself. I feel suffocated." In a way, Fawn was running from herself when she unknowingly tried to run from her broken heart. Unfortunately, we cannot run or hide from our broken hearts. Unlike a broken leg that can be amputated, our hearts cannot be fixed the same way. Even if our untreated grief causes damage to our physical hearts and we replace them through a heart transplant, they would remain broken and in pain if not treated appropriately.

Maxwell Maltz, in his book *Self-Image Psychology*, describes a woman who got a scar on her face secondary to an event that shattered her life and her emotional heart.[6] Even after her facial scar was removed and repaired beautifully through plastic surgery, this woman did not feel any better. Even though she looked better, she did not feel better because her damaged self-image and the associated grief from her shattered life and heart had not been resolved.

We cannot run or hide from our grief when our emotional hearts are broken because it is as if a meteor has entered a dormant volcano. Upon impact, the hot lava in the shaken volcano flows into every crevice inside it. The grief that comes from our tough time is like this hot lava inside of us. Imagine running around with hot lava flowing inside of you. You cannot run away from something inside of you. In fact, the more you try to run away, the more you feel the pain and pressure from the heat. The more you try to run away from your grief, the more you feel its pain and pressure. This is why Fawn started to feel suffocated as she unknowingly tried to run from her grief.

We cannot run from the grief inside of us because it will seep into our system and cause more damage. We cannot put it on the shelf either because it will flow over and catch up with us. Instead, we want to clear it out through the guidance of professionals.

The Turmoil of Thoughts

Fawn said, "I can't stop thinking now … I think I am just crazy to be more in pain now when I should feel much better."

It is sad, but not surprising, that Fawn's "thinking and thinking" did not help her feel any better—when we have a broken heart, we grieve, and grief has everything to do with feeling, and very little to do with thinking. In fact, using our intellect is not helpful when we want to heal our broken hearts because thinking and trying to make sense of our feelings can often cause us to be more confused and cause us to feel more pain.

Have you ever heard something that makes sense intellectually but didn't make you feel any better? For example, when Roscoe, my twenty-year-old cat, died and my neighbor told me, "He had a good long life already," logically, I knew it was great that Roscoe lived until twenty, but I didn't care. Emotionally, I felt devastated. I wanted him to live longer. I felt sad, scared, confused, and discouraged by all the grief-ridden events in my life. I felt irritated by my neighbor's comment, even though I knew she was right: Roscoe had lived a good life.

Since grief has everything to do with feeling, it is important to identify our feelings in order to be able to navigate and move through (and beyond) our grief for two reasons. The first reason is: if we are unaware that what we are experiencing are feelings instead of thoughts, we will try to approach our feelings as if they are our thoughts. We judge our feelings as either rational or irrational, as right or wrong. If we think our feelings (confused for thoughts) are irrational or wrong, we feel bad, despite there being no right or wrong, logical or illogical feelings. We feel bad on top of our present state of grief, which then leads us to feel worse. This was evident as Fawn started to feel that she was wrong and crazy even though it was completely normal.

The second reason it is important to put our thinking cap aside when we are grieving is that grief has everything to do with feelings and very little to do with thinking.[1] The more we try to think about it, the more confused we become. We try to make sense of something that is not meant to be made sense of, and as a result, we feel totally lost.

When we are grieving, it is as if we have been dropped into a convoluted maze equipped with obstacles made of feelings. For us to be able to emerge safely from our labyrinth of unpleasant feelings, we want to first recognize these obstacles so that we can clear them out of our path. If we are unaware that what we are experiencing are feelings and we focus only on our thinking, not only are we not clearing the "feeling obstacles," but we often end up deeper in our maze of misery—just as Fawn did. Fawn said, "I can't stop thinking … thinking maybe I did something wrong that made me lose my baby, thinking maybe I was guilty of something in the past and this is the punishment … crazy to be more in pain now." Fawn ended up with her thoughts running wild in her maze of misery.

Unfortunately, it is not always easy to know whether we are feeling or thinking about something. Many of us confuse feeling with thinking because, growing up in this modern society, we are trained by our society to think rather than feel. Most schools don't teach us much about feelings, never mind noticing, honoring, and navigating our feelings. Many people say that they "think" something when they are actually feeling it.

One way to know whether you are feeling or thinking something is to see if you can replace the word "think" with "feel" in your sentence. If your sentence still makes sense even after you replace the word "think" with "feel" without adding any other words, then it is a feeling that you are experiencing, and there is no right or wrong, good or bad feeling.

We want to endeavor to recognize, acknowledge, and honor our feelings, and, as much as we can, let go of our "thinking cap" when we are navigating through grief. Too much thinking when our hearts are broken will put us in even more emotional turmoil. We will not be perfect in our endeavor, but as we discussed in the first chapter, perfection is never the goal. We do the best we can, and we must not allow ourselves to think that we are not good enough.

Hung by a string of Gs

G is for Guilty.

Guilt and grief are like two best buddies that seem inseparable. Practically everyone who experiences grief carries with them a string of guilt. A client, Natasha, had the guilt of not visiting her grandfather on his very last birthday because she had the flu and did not want to risk passing the illness on to him. Unfortunately, her grandfather unexpectedly passed away two days after his birthday. Natasha, who conducts a very healthy lifestyle, also felt guilty that she had the flu during such an unfortunate time. She suspected she caught the flu during a long flight for a work trip. In her turmoil of overthinking, she felt she should have somehow known that her grandfather would die unexpectedly two days after his eightieth birthday, and that she should have known that going on the work trip would have been a mistake. Or perhaps she should have taken shorter connecting flights or worn a mask during the flights.

Some people even feel guilty about things that contradict each other. In my own journey with Roscoe's death, I felt guilty for not brushing his fur earlier that week and having him look nicer when he died. He hated having his fur brushed, so I also felt guilty for insisting on brushing him every other week during the last year of his life to keep his coat and skin healthy.

Some of us feel guilty when our well-intentioned friends indirectly suggest that there could be a reason for us to feel guilty, such as with Fawn. Looking back, Fawn recalled a friend who said "You should not feel guilty. It's not your fault at all that you had a miscarriage." Unfortunately, this type of comment almost always causes grievers to question themselves and eventually believe that they are guilty. This happens to such an extent that when we cannot see apparent wrongdoings on which to blame ourselves, we start looking around to see if there is something else for which we are guilty. We start to overthink everything, and we get trapped in a turmoil of thoughts as a result.

Why are we so inclined to feel guilty when disaster happens? One explanation for this guilt complex is that, in truth, most of us really want to do our best but end up feeling inadequate when we don't reach that standard. The epidemic of feeling "not good enough" is so prevalent that we often label people who do not suffer from this complex as arrogant or even narcissistic. The true definition of a narcissist is a person who has an excessive interest in or admiration of themselves, and whose symptoms impair one or more aspects of their lives.[7] This combination of wanting to do our best but feeling "not good enough" is a recipe for feeling wrong in our actions, which thereby leads to the feeling of guilt.

"Guilt," according to the Merriam-Webster online dictionary, is the "feeling of deserving blame, especially for imagined offenses or from a sense of inadequacy." The Free Dictionary online says that guilt is a painful emotion experienced when one believes that one's actions or thoughts have violated a moral or personal standard. We feel guilty because we have a concept of how we could have affected things that were not within our control, such as the sudden passing of a grandfather.

We feel guilty when, in truth, most of us have no valid reason to feel guilty at all. Guilt, according to Dictionary. com, is the fact or state of having committed an offense, crime, violation, or wrong, especially against moral or penal law. Unless you truly have committed a crime or intentionally done something to hurt someone, you do not have any real guilt. Knowing that our guilty feelings arise from a concept in our minds regarding how we wished things could be, we can let go of our feelings of guilt.

We can now let go of our guilty feelings by recognizing that, in most cases, the guilty feelings we have are actually our desire that things had happened differently or that we had known better in the moment, even if there was no way for us to have known otherwise.

We might wish things could have been different, and we might be devastated by our tragedy, but it is not our fault that things happened the way they did. It was not Natasha's fault that her grandfather died suddenly, nor was it Fawn's fault that she had a miscarriage, nor was it my fault that Roscoe disliked getting brushed. However, it is our choice and our responsibility to stop letting our guilty feelings strangle us while we are navigating through our grief.

We can experience grief without also being hung by a string of guilt. We can recognize and acknowledge that we are in a maze of grief and that the guilty feelings are obstacle blocks that we can now remove.

The "F" Word

"F" is for "Forgiving." Now, before you decided to skip reading this whole section, please know that you are not being asked to approve, agree to, tolerate, or forget any wrongdoing done by anybody, including yourself.

"F" is for "Forgiving." Listen to the word. It sounds so much like "to give for." Give away the old clothes so that we can have space for new and better ones. Give away things that do not make us feel good for things that give us peace of mind, ease, and joy. Give away old drinking or smoking habits so that we can live a full, healthy life. Give away and let go of our old baggage of anger, resentment, and guilt so that we can have ease, peace of mind, love, and joy. Let go of our memories of what happened in the past for a more peaceful mind and heart with which to fully recover from our heartbreak.

To forgive is to stop letting our memories of a past event continue to ruin our lives in the present and future.[8] Forgiving has nothing to do with approving, making right, condoning, agreeing, or even tolerating any wrongdoing, including things that you believe that you yourself could have done differently in the past.

69

Forgiving is like getting rid of a malignant tumor on our bodies. All malignant tumors have toxic roots penetrating deep and wide into the places where they grow. What we see on our bodies is only the tip of the iceberg of the tumor. We can cut off the tumor, but if we do not clear out the body of the iceberg, the toxic roots of the tumor will continue to do harm. If left untreated, these roots often grow a new tumor. Even worse, if left untreated, these toxic, malignant roots will continue to penetrate deeper and further and start spreading their toxic, malignant cells into the whole body. Then the tumor spreads and may eventually kill us.

Having resentment, guilt, shame, or anger is like having a malignant tumor in our lives. We want to clear out the resentment and anger that we have toward others. However, this alone is not enough, for resentment and anger are often only the tip of the iceberg. We want to clear out the toxic, malignant roots of the tumor of our lives as well, the ones that can cause more damage than the tumor itself. One clue that we still have toxic, malignant roots to clear out is that we hear ourselves saying, "I wish I had not…" or "I could have…" or "Why didn't (or did) I…" We want to release our guilt, shame, and self-blame, as these can rob us of our peace of mind and cause even worse emotional and psychological damage than anger and resentment. Until we forgive our opponents and ourselves, we will continue to be chained to the 100-pound ball of our past. Until we can break the chain that weighs us down and learn how to forgive, it will be very difficult for us to be able to fully move on with our lives.

Forgiveness is a multilayered process and often takes time. Some of us forgive quickly and easily; some have difficulty even starting to forgive. Do not get discouraged if you find it difficult to forgive a very painful event. The first and most important step is that you are willing to forgive. Do not get discouraged if you have been carrying your emotional cancer for decades. It is never too late to start taking steps to forgiveness.

To forgive is to give ourselves peace of mind, joy, and the ability to fully move on. To forgive is to move forward to the point where nothing from our past interactions still disturb us. Yet, some of us still choose not to even try to forgive. That's okay; it is your choice not to forgive. It is your choice to continue to feel the pang of anger. It is your choice to continue to hold on to your memories that do nothing but bring you pain. It is your choice not to have true freedom of mind and heart. It is okay if you do not want to even try to forgive now—because the opportunity will always be available. When you are ready, the opportunity to forgive will still be there.

NEW BEGINNING

Forget-Me-Not

Don, a newcomer to the Dance Away Sadness: Move Beyond Your Grief community class, waited until everyone else had left before he came to speak with me. "Thank you for the class. It really helped me to move some sadness that I didn't know I still had after ten years."

"You're very welcome. I'm glad it helped. What happened ten years ago? Is there anything else I can do to help you?" I asked.

He hesitated and then said, "I lost my wife to cancer. What's your thought on moving on and, um, remarrying?"

"I think it is fine to move on and to remarry if that's what you want to do, and if not, that's fine too."

Don quickly replied, "No, I don't want to do that; I don't want to betray her. My adult kids want me to date again and to move on, because I get lonely. They said that their mom told me to remarry after she died, but don't you think that's being unfaithful to her?"

"No," I said. "You are not at all being unfaithful to her by moving on and dating again, or even remarrying. You are expressing your love to her and honoring her by moving on, if that is something that also makes you happy. You see, when you truly love someone, you want them to be happy. Even after their passing, the ones who truly love us want us to be able to have peace of mind and happiness, not to live with sadness, anger, loneliness, or regret. So, you are actually honoring your late wife's wish when you are able to move on and live a fulfilling life again, even if she had not asked you to remarry before her passing." I paused to see if he had any questions.

Don thought about it, "Okay. But I love her, and I don't want to forget her."

"Don, you will not forget your late wife. We will

not forget someone whom we truly love, whether that person be a spouse, a child, or a pet. The difference is, when you're able to move on, you can remember your late wife without feeling pain and sadness.[1] Almost everyone, including our loved ones, wants to be loved and remembered in a cherished way. Even after you move on, you'll still remember your wife and cherish the fun memories you had with her. When you are able to move, you are actually expressing your love to her."

Don nodded, "You're right. Thank you. I feel so much better now. It'll be good to not live in such a big, empty house, alone and lonely. The kids will be happy, and I'll feel better too. Do you have any advice for me on moving on?"

"One thing is to remember that even after you move on, it is normal to have moments of sadness still. It is common and normal to miss our loved ones on special dates or random moments. As our hearts heal and we recover from our grief, we will feel less sadness. Just as everyone has different fingerprints, everyone takes a different amount of time to heal and move on. It is quite normal to feel that you are moving three steps forward and two steps back. Just be patient with yourself, and don't expect to do things perfectly. It also helps to practice gratitude. It helps you to focus on what's good and to stay calm."

No Spiritual Bypass

This time Don looked doubtful. "Gratitude? Hmmm,

there's nothing about losing my wife to nasty cancer to be grateful for."

"No. Of course not," I said. "I don't imagine so, and I am not asking you to be grateful for that. However, there are many other things in life that we can be grateful for even when something undesirable has happened. We are not grateful that our loved one died or that the house burned down, but we can be grateful for other things that we have taken for granted, like having a roof over our heads.

"Our gratitude is not meant to be a spiritual bypass for things that cause our heartbreak. We want to express gratitude for other things in our lives that are still going well, because in addition to the emotional/psychological benefits, expressing gratitude also has physical benefits. It causes a release in dopamine that lowers our heart rate, reduces anxiety and depression, and helps us to relax. Expressing gratitude also stimulates our hypothalamus, and thus helps us sleep better."

Don nodded again. "I see what you mean. I am grateful to have found your Dance Away Sadness class and to be learning from you. What other tips do you have for me to be able to move on?"

"I am grateful that you took the bold step to continue recovering from your wife's death. There are many other tools and skills I can share for being able to move beyond your grief and thrive. One very important thing is to have a 'forward fortitude attitude,' which is a set of skills that allows us to have ease and peace of mind even as we are going through a tough time." We'll discuss this in more detail in the next chapter.

REVIEW

1. You are NOT broken. You have a broken heart, but you are whole and courageous.
2. Passing time and staying busy do not heal.
3. Grief and a broken heart are "feeling" matters. Overthinking and overanalyzing will exacerbate and add to our grief.
4. Guilt is a feeling that comes from an expectation that we have for ourselves. It is okay not to feel guilty.
5. Forgiveness has nothing to do with agreeing or approving. It is to let go of the memories that continue to ruin our current lives.
6. Moving on is honoring and an expression of our love to our loved one.
7. Gratitude is not a spiritual bypass.

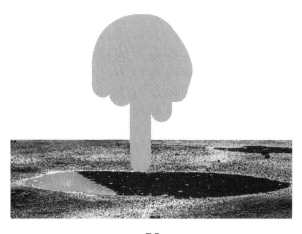

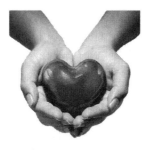

Chapter 4

FORWARD FORTITUDE

T he French eat a lot more red-meat than Americans or the British, and they have fewer heart attacks.

The Italians drink a lot more red wine than Americans or the British, and they, too, have fewer heart attacks.

The Japanese smoke a lot more cigarettes than Americans or the British, but they, too, have fewer heart attacks.

The conclusion is clear: eat or drink whatever you want; it is speaking English that kills you![9]

The fourth step for navigating through our disasters and their associated grief comes from our fourth finger. We use our fourth finger to help us remember to continue to move forth despite all the adversity that we are experiencing. Take these steps imperfectly but with the best attitude, knowing that one baby step at a time will take us up and over any mountain.

Our fourth finger helps us remember to be a person with forward fortitude and to have courage in the face of adversity. Understanding grief and having a two-thumbs-up attitude will help us move through grief and recover completely. Possessing forward fortitude with gratitude will help make our journey easier and faster. Practicing forward fortitude will help us recover and thrive after our life has fallen apart. In this chapter, we will discuss the skills and tools that will help us to continue moving forward with a positive attitude, even as we navigate through our tough time.

THE SKY FALLS AGAIN

A Date at the MRI

"Pretend you're happy when you're blue, it isn't very hard … and nothing's as bad as it may seem." The wonderful voice of Nat King Cole came out from the speakers in the neurologist's office as I sat all alone in the waiting room on a Friday evening, waiting for yet another urgent MRI. What a song to play in a neurologist's office! "Are they playing this song intentionally?" I wondered. I was not sure if I should cry or laugh when I heard the song, because I did feel "blue." I did not plan on having a date with an MRI machine on a Friday evening, nor did I ever dream of suddenly losing the strength and function of my right hand. In less than two weeks, I went from having a perfectly functioning, normal right hand to having difficulty in performing my tasks at work, writing, putting my clothes on, and eating.

I saw the life that I had rebuilt with sweat and tears over the last eight years crumbling rapidly in front of my very eyes. All the costly tests could not identify the cause of my hand and arm problem, and the neurologist could not treat it either. I was facing a handicap, losing my job for which I went to school for twenty-five years, and losing my ability to take care of my parents and myself. Out of the blue, my sky was falling again. The song kept on going, "Just close your eyes…"

I closed my eyes and took a deep breath. I chose to laugh at the irony of having a neurologist's office play this song late on a Friday evening, and thought of something about my situation that I could be grateful for. It is surely not my preference to be having an MRI—my third MRI in a week, at 8 pm on Friday evening—but at least I was able to have all these MRIs and tests at a moment's notice. I am very grateful for having both the financial abundance and great health insurance to be able to do these tests. Also, after having been through at least eight tragedies in two years and witnessing others do the same, I know that in most cases "Nothing's as bad as it may seem…" just as the song said. Even if it is, there's a seed of equal or greater good in every adversity, every heartbreak, and every failure, as Napoleon Hill said.

I took another deep breath and opened my eyes, just

at the right time to see an elderly couple come out from the MRI area with a young man in a wheelchair. I could see smeared mascara and dry tears on the woman's face. The young man who was secured to the wheelchair had a thick bandage wrapped around his head, and he was drooping to one side with uncontrollable twitching on that side. Surely, my problem was not remotely as bad as theirs. I was very grateful that I was in much better shape than he was.

The trio left the neurologist's waiting room, and I was all alone again. Out of the blue, my thoughts and fears started up again. "You think you are in better shape than that guy. How do you know you are not going to end up like him? You are having a problem with your right hand and arm now, so how do you know it's not going to spread until you are paralyzed? Three top doctors can't figure out what's going on with you; how do you know you are not going to become quadriplegic? How do you know you won't lose your job soon, and you and your parents won't become homeless because you are the only child and you are supposed to take care of them? Your boyfriend will leave you because he won't want a quadriplegic woman. You might as well kill yourself…"

"STOP! PAUSE! None of these horror stories are happening right now, so we are not talking about them." I stomped my foot to silence the fearful thoughts. I am grateful that in my journey of learning to thrive after my previous disasters and heartbreak, I have learned to notice my thoughts and my moods and to stop the destructive ones. The receptionist noticed my stomping and said, "Sorry for the long wait. The one just now took a bit longer than we thought it would."

What nice people, I thought. They had fit me in and stayed at work late, and now they were apologizing for the wait. "Oh no! Don't worry about the wait," I replied quickly. "I just had, err, a little cramp in my leg. Thank you for fitting me in. I hope I'm not ruining your Friday night plans too much."

The receptionist smiled and said cheerfully, "Not at all. I don't make any plans on Thursday and Friday evenings in case we need to stay late. It's life, and things happen, you know."

"The guy just now looked like he was in bad shape," I said, referring to the young man in the wheelchair.

The receptionist nodded. "Yes, it's very sad. He was standing on the sidewalk outside of their home, and a drunk driver hit him."

"Oh dear! That's horrible!" I exclaimed.

She nodded, "It is. We never know about life; we just have to make the best of the time we have."

"We just have to make the best of the time we have here on earth. Be happy and grateful for what we have now," I echoed, and started paying closer attention to my surroundings to see what else I could be grateful for.

I noticed a wall mural of a sunny day on a little Italian street. There was a café on the street with a colorful awning and windows lined with lovely, joyful, and colorful flowers in window beds. Two women were sitting at the table outside the café; the one whose face was visible was smiling. I chose to smile back at her; I smiled and felt a little less tense. Now, I could almost feel myself standing there, smelling the lovely aroma from the café and feeling the Mediterranean sun on my skin. I chose to allow myself to savor the lovely feeling of my imagination at work so that I could feel even a little more relaxed. Now, I felt I could lower my shoulder.

I looked back at the reception area and noticed the orchids. There was one orchid plant on each of the three counters and two on the shelf behind the receptionist. I love orchids, so my head must have really been stuck in the sand of fear and self-pity for me not to have noticed them. They remind me of my favorite grandmother, who I know still looks after me even after she passed away long ago. I allowed myself to feel supported by my late grandmother, knowing that she would not abandon my parents and me, and I felt a little more at peace.

I looked at the other wall of the waiting room. There were beautiful life-sized poster panels. Altogether, they painted a vivid image of families playing in the sand on a sunny day at the beach. It was so vivid that I could almost hear the children laughing and feel their happiness. I chose to embrace their joy and allow myself to chuckle a little. I am so happy and grateful for this happy painting, and I noticed my heart felt lighter as the clouds lifted from my mind.

The observant receptionist noticed my change in mood and said with a big smile, "Aren't they just lovely posters? I look at them whenever I feel blue, and they help me feel better. Oh, and the MRI technician just told me that they are ready for you. She is coming out to get you now."

The MRI technician was polite, but she seemed to be a little tense and distant. I chose to be friendly, joyful, and appreciative regardless. I thanked her for staying late and fitting me in. She relaxed a little, "No problem. Just doing my job."

"Thank you for doing your job so wonderfully, even at this late hour. I really appreciate your dedication to helping your patients," I replied with genuine appreciation and a big, friendly smile. She smiled too.

"Oh, thank you. I appreciate it. And yes, of course, we are here to help. Here's your gown. Let's have you use this bigger bathroom to change. Then you can put your belongings in this lockbox. And take your time, I'm here for you." She smiled and looked noticeably more relaxed.

I changed quickly while noticing the lovely floral decor and big, beautiful crystal chandeliers on the ceiling of the hallway around the MRI machine. I told the MRI technician, "It's so pretty in here. It feels almost like I'm in a fine restaurant."

She chuckled, "Well, we know the patients are already stressed, so the management tries to make it as pleasant as possible in here. I've never heard any patient say that, though." She chuckled again. "I think most people don't even notice. Most people are too drowned in their own thoughts and worries, which I understand."

The words of Eleanor Roosevelt came to my mind, and I paraphrased them out loud: "All the water in the world cannot drown you if you do not let it get into you."

The MRI technician nodded, "That's true. You are going to be in the machine for about two hours. We can have a break halfway through if you need it. Are you okay with that?"

"Yes, I am, thank you. I'll have a lovely date with the MRI machine in this beautiful restaurant of life for the next two hours or so," I said cheerfully. The previously tense and distant MRI technician laughed.

"And I'll be your server for your date. Just press the buzzer in your hand if you need anything."

My intimate date with the MRI machine went very smoothly, and the two hours flew by. "Thank you again for staying late and fitting me in," I said to my new friend the MRI technician.

She looked at me and said: "Thank you for being so nice. I've done this for fifteen years, and you are the nicest and most relaxed patient I have had. Most people are so stressed and grumpy even if they are just coming in for a quick MRI before a routine ACL surgery. I hope the doctors figure out what's going on with your hand and arm so that they can treat you properly. I know everything will work out well for you since you have such good energy." I thanked her and, perhaps coincidentally, as I left the neurologist's office, the music played Israel Kamakawiwo: "Somewhere over the rainbow, bluebirds fly ... the clouds are far behind, and troubles melt like lemon drops."

Yes, eventually all storms will stop, and a beautiful rainbow comes out afterward. It is up to us to cry when the sky first falls, but then to either safely sing and dance in the rain or scream and mope through the whole storm. It is also up to us to look up at the fresh sky once the storm stops so that we can see the rainbow. We will only see it if we remember to look up at the fresh sky after the storm. Paraphrasing Eleanor Roosevelt again, "All the storm and water in the world cannot drown us if we do not let it get into us."

Hopes Unmet

"I'm so sorry. I'm so sorry for everything you've been through in the last four months. From your right hand and arm having problems, to your parents' health problems, and now your breakup. I'm so sorry. It must be very tough on you. Let me know if I can help," Ana, my housecleaner, said to me when she learned that my boyfriend of seven years and I were no longer together romantically.

"Oh, thank you. Thank you for offering to help. Yes, it has been a very rough few months," I admitted.

Ana was right. As if the peculiar time-and-money-consuming, life-altering problem with my right hand and arm were not enough, a couple of months later, my mother suddenly grew ill. Now my long-term boyfriend and I decided to end our romantic relationship. Even though we continued to stay friends, I was still heartbroken. I loved this man very much. We had lots of fun together; he introduced me to life's adventures and passions that I didn't even know could be possible. He helped me to heal my broken heart and was my greatest cheerleader as I rebuilt my broken life. I thought back to the first time I allowed myself to be flown away for a long weekend trip without knowing where we were going. He was the first man with whom I felt completely safe. He was very genuine, smart, wise, and kind. We were a great sounding board for each other, and at the same time, a very soft shoulder for each other to cry on. Now all these things had to change. Yes, we ended our relationship on great terms and continued to be friends. Yes, we would continue to be each other's cheerleaders, sounding boards, and soft places to fall. No, it was not going to be the same anymore. No, we would not be growing old together.

Not only did I lose a boyfriend and all the security and routine of that relationship, but I also lost all my hopes and dreams for our future together. The Grief Recovery Institute calls this "loss of unmet hopes and dreams." It adds another layer of grief to the initial loss itself. It is a concept that is quite easy to understand. Yet, understanding it does not make it any easier. Understanding it does not change the fact that I was looking at my sky falling yet again.

On the other hand, my grief felt different this time. Even with everything that went on back then, I did not have the risk of losing my ability to work in a career that I had dedicated my life to so far. This career had become my identity, one that had been my safety net, my joy, and my pride. My mother's illness complicated my situation even more, as I never had to take the risk of not having her around for support before. This time, there was even more uncertainty and unmet hopes in addition to heartbreak.

Yet, I felt different this time. This time, I felt very calm. This time, I had moments of sadness, but I was genuinely happy the other 95 percent of the time. This time, I had moments of worry, but they were hardly as prevalent or overwhelming as they were eight years ago, even though my future was still at risk as long as there was no solution for my hand and arm problem. This time, my former boyfriend and I remained supportive friends instead of the strangers that my former husband and I had become. This time, I remained joyful despite my bleeding heart after the end of my relationship with my former boyfriend. This time, I was looking at possibly losing my mother and the life that I had worked very hard to make for myself, but I continued to be grateful.

My friends, coworkers, clients, parents, and former boyfriend regularly and consistently told me that I looked and sounded just fine. I remained grateful and maintained my happy and calm self, despite having one heartbreaking tragedy after another. How could I consistently be happy, joyful, grateful, and at peace during such an uncertain time? How was it that I was not experiencing nearly as much confusion, fear, despair, and anger this time? Was I in denial? Was I being a Pollyanna, naively optimistic? Had I gotten very good at pretending to be happy? No, it was none of these things; it was practicing forward-fortitude with gratitude even in the face of grievous circumstances.

FORWARD-FORTITUDE

Fortitude is courage in the face of pain or adversity. It is the strength to bear misfortune and pain, calmly and patiently.

Having forward-fortitude is choosing to continue taking one step forward at a time despite all the adversity that we are experiencing—and doing it with the best attitude we can possibly have. It is gratitude for what is still good, despite unpleasant circumstances. It is also doing these things imperfectly.

Forward-fortitude with gratitude is not faking it, or pretending, or denying, or being a Pollyanna. Forward-fortitude is chosen optimism with action. It is being fully aware that the glass is half empty, being grateful that the glass is half full, exploring what can be done to have the glass completely refilled with sparkling water, and doing whatever it is that can be done promptly, albeit imperfectly.

Acknowledging, honoring, and understanding grief and having a two-thumbs-up attitude helps us to navigate through our grief and recover from it fully. Practicing forward-fortitude with gratitude is the piece of the puzzle that allows the journey to be a lot smoother, easier, faster, and more fruitful. There are several tools and skills that are keys in having forward-fortitude with gratitude, in choosing to be an optimist with gratitude.

Is the Beach Ball Red or Green?

Our first tool for being a person with forward-fortitude is the tool of perception.

Have you ever seen one of those huge multicolored beach balls? Imagine you are standing very closely in front of a giant, house-sized, multicolored beach ball and you are wearing a pair of dark sunglasses. What colors do you see? Perhaps dark red? Or murky blue? Now imagine another person standing across from you on the opposite side of this giant beach ball. What color might that person see? Perhaps it is the same color as you see, or perhaps a different color altogether. Now imagine that I ask you and the other person to tell me one color you see on this giant beach ball. In other words, you cannot say it is multicolored even if you think it might be multicolored. Would you call out the color you see in front of you? The other person would likely do the same. If each of you were calling out a different color, would one of you be incorrect? No, you would both be correct, as you called out the color you could see. Now imagine that you removed your dark sunglasses while continuing to look at this giant beach ball. Would it still look the same, or brighter?

This is perception. Just as our ability to see brightness clearly is highly influenced by the clarity of our lens, our ability to think clearly is greatly influenced by the clarity of our mind. When a disaster happens and we are grieving, the state of our perception can be compared to wearing a pair of dark sunglasses: everything seems darker and murkier than it might actually be. Just as our ability to see physical things is limited by the quality of our eyesight, our perception of dire circumstances is limited by the depth of our awareness and understanding of life.

Now imagine you took a couple of steps back away from the ball—you would then see the ball from an entirely different perspective. Rather than seeing only blue, you would see all the colors that create this beautiful, giant beach ball. We can do the same when we are in dire circumstances. We can remove our dark sunglasses and take a couple of steps away to detach ourselves from the circumstances. When we do this, we often see that what had appeared to be a murky blue situation is part of a colorful circle of life. Once we see the whole circle, we clearly see the way to resolve our circumstances by either going around the ball or over it.

Being able to have a broader perception of our circumstances will allow us to see more clearly. We will realize that most things are not as bad as they seem, and even when it is bad, there will be ways around it. Like the beach ball that could not be seen for its true beauty until viewed from far away, there are goods that we are not able to see when we are fighting through our circumstances. What we want to do is to detach ourselves from our circumstances in order to see the bigger picture. As Napoleon Hill said, "There is a seed of equal or greater good in every adversity, every failure, and every heartbreak." It is up to us to remember that we need the nighttime before we can have a beautiful sunrise.

The Nine-Second Master-Move

Our second tool for being a person with forward-fortitude is practicing the nine-second master-move. If we practice this move along with the other tools in this chapter, we will become masters of our emotions.

"STOP! *PAUSE!* None of these horror stories are happening right now, so we are not talking about it now." I stomped my foot and silently ordered my fearful thoughts away the moment I noticed that my mind was going toward the dark abyss as I sat waiting at the neurologist's office.

Notice

The first part of our nine-second master-move is to notice. Notice what's running through our minds, what's boiling in our emotional hearts, and any internal whirlwind that we might be experiencing at the moment. As Mary Morrissey, the award-winning author and founder of DreamBuilder, says: "Notice what you're noticing." Noticing our thoughts and our feelings is crucial in being able to have forward-fortitude with gratitude. We want to be able to notice when we have frightening thoughts or catastrophic feelings about the worst potential outcome of our circumstances. Why? Because we need to first notice our feelings and thoughts before we can decide whether they are empowering to us or not. We must notice before we can stop and replace the disempowering thoughts and feelings with something more empowering to us. In other words, we cannot choose to have thoughts and feelings that are more empowering if we don't know what's running through our minds and our emotions.

Pause

The second part of our nine-second master-move is to pause any thoughts and feelings that are not serving us. We push our internal pause button as soon as we notice any internal turmoil, and choose between letting our internal whirlwind take us for a ride or becoming the master of our own thoughts and emotions.

Choose

The third part of our nine-second master-move is to choose. It is completely up to us, and we are the only ones who can choose between keeping or replacing the negative thoughts and feelings that harm us. Just as there is no right or wrong feeling, there is no right or wrong choice. It is just as "right" to want to keep our dark sunglasses on while attaching ourselves to the giant beach ball of obstacles as it is to take our dark sunglasses off and take a couple of steps back so that we can see clearly and think more productively. It is completely up to us to choose better over bitter, practice forward-fortitude with gratitude, move beyond our disaster, and thrive. The moment we notice our internal turmoil and push our internal pause button, we can decide to replace the "fear-anger-worry-doubt-despair" with something else more empowering.

Decide

The fourth and final step in our nine-second master-move is to decide. We must decide that we are going to replace disempowering thoughts and feelings with ones that take us a step closer to thriving after our disaster. We must decide that we will let go and be better instead of bitter. Even more importantly, we must decide that we are going to do what it takes to be, and stay, more empowered, to have less internal turmoil, to have more peace of mind, to recover fully and completely, to thrive even after our sky has crumbled on us, and to live joyfully again.

These four fundamental steps are the most important and powerful tools we have for being able to recover from and move beyond our tragedy. All together, these four steps take less than nine seconds, but if we endeavor to practice them regularly and consistently while we are navigating through our daily life, this nine-second master-move will bring us decades of life with more ease and joy. What is your decision?

Breathe in the Simple Present

Have you ever felt overwhelmed? Have you ever worried? Do you ever have regrets?

Our third tool for being a person with forward-fortitude is a bundle of three keys that are very effective in helping us to worry less and feel less overwhelmed. These keys are: notice our breathing, focus on the present, and simplify our life as much as we can.

Just Breathe

When was the last time you really noticed your breathing?

One of the simplest, fastest, free, doable-at-any-moment tools for feeling less overwhelmed is to notice our breathing. Simply notice our inhales and our exhales. We do not have to take a few cycles of deep breaths if it is not convenient to do so, simply notice our inhales and exhales.

Just noticing our breathing for a few breaths and sending gratitude to our system will actually calm and relax us. Even if we are in the midst of an overwhelming conversation, we can simply notice our inhales and exhales without feeling awkward or causing a distraction to the persons with whom we are speaking. What do you notice about your breathing at this very moment? If you notice that you are breathing fast and shallow right now, you can choose to breathe deeper and slower to help you relax.

What about deep breathing or meditation? If you are in a place where you can perform several cycles of deep breathing or meditation, you may do that as well. Studies have clearly shown that deep breathing and meditation decrease our heart rate and blood pressure and increase our theta brain waves.[10] An increase in our theta brain wave activity causes us to be more creative and come up with solutions to our problems. You may refer to the appendix section of this book for more deep breathing techniques. However, if you are not at a place where you can practice deep breathing, just noticing your breathing for two or three cycles will immediately help you feel calmer and reduce your anxiety. Let's try noticing our breathing more this week, perhaps before we go to bed, and see if we notice any difference in how we feel after one week.

Simple Present

Did you know that, unlike the English, French, or Spanish languages that have past, present, and future tenses, the Indonesian language only has one tense? The Indonesian language only has the present tense, and it adds a time connotation to talk about the past or the future. Having only the present tense makes the Indonesian language a lot easier.

One of the shortest well-known quotes from Henry David Thoreau is: "Simplify, simplify, simplify." Following this quote in his essay "Walden," Thoreau said, "We do not ride the railroad; it rides upon us."[11] Nowadays, that railroad is often our smartphone and the many other electronics that we use in our lives. Living in this modern world, we often acquire so many things to have and do that they end up bogging down our lives. We end up running in a hamster wheel of trying to get, have, and do more.

One of the best tools for having less to worry about is to be as simple as possible in the present. Be present in the present and simplify what we can simplify. If you can, simplify your daily routine to something that's much simpler that also feels good to you. Focus on who and what you really love, and let go of what is not crucial. Be present in the present, let go of the "what if," and focus on the "what *is*." Many times, we try to speculate on what might happen and then try to prepare for something that won't necessarily happen. Just the thought of having to do this can make us feel overwhelmed.

We will be more at ease and accomplish our tasks more efficiently when we let go of the future tense and stay with the present tense. Take care of what we can care for now, and do so in the simplest way possible. Take just one simple step at a time. Try not to become so anxious and overwhelmed about what the future might hold that we don't slow ourselves down now or, even worse, end up with an illness in our physical bodies from our anxiety. Let's take care of the most crucial matter that is right in front of us in the most direct and simple way possible and, before long, we will take care of everything that needs to be addressed—and we'll do it with more ease.

Staying in the present can also help us to move beyond our regrets. Let go of what was and focus on what is. When we have regrets, we tend to think about the past and wish that we had done things differently. The fact is that we did the best we could at the given moment. Feeling guilty will only make us feel horrible; it will not reverse the past, nor will it improve the future. Let's instead focus on the present. What one or more lessons have we learned from the experience? What one simple thing can we do now, based on the lessons we have learned, so that we do not repeat the past? Let's let go of "what was" and focus on "what is."

Let's let go of the past tense and the future tense and focus on the simple present tense.

NATO with Gratitude

Our fourth tool for being a person with forward-fortitude is to practice NATO with gratitude.

Buddha said, "All life is suffering. The cause of suffering is attachment." I once met a wise and very successful older gentleman who told me that his secret of living a peaceful, joyful life was that he learned to only "prefer" instead of "need."

"You know, Birgitte, you can learn to practice NATO (No Attachment to Outcome) with gratitude. You can have a strong preference, but no attachment. When you must have something or someone, you become closely attached to it and afraid of losing it, so you anxiously start to cling to it. Do you want anyone to cling to you or grip you tightly all the time? It is repulsive to have someone anxiously cling to or grip you, isn't it? On the other hand, when you prefer something, you welcome it. You still do the best that you can to bring forth what you very much prefer, but if it does not happen, you have not gone through the anxiety and the suffering. You are grateful for, and make the best of, what you have for now, and know that something better is on its way if you stay positive."

The wise old man smiled as he waved his hand toward the grand balcony over his waterfall and palm tree-lined Olympic-sized swimming pool that appeared to merge with the ocean in front of it and said, "A lot of people get to where I am in life with so much stress that it almost kills them because they are always fighting. They fight for their must-haves, and once they have them, they become too afraid of losing them. It is unhealthy how they are tense and worried all the time. I just relax, stay very focused on my preference, and do the very best that I can every time. I do not worry about things. I hold everything with open hands and an open heart, even during tough times. I have a lot more peace and fun in life, I stay healthier because I have less stress, and people find me very pleasant, which further helps me in my work. That's the secret for which you are asking, Birgitte, the secret for having been through so much, become so successful, and having remained light-hearted and tranquil. When tough times happen, do the very best that you can in order to make the best of what you have, and for the things you can't change, do your best to accept them while trying to find the seed of greater good. You do all these with open hands, an open heart, and gratitude. Be grateful for what you still have." He looked at me to see if I had captured his teaching.

I nodded in accordance. "Practice NATO, No Attachment to Outcome, with gratitude, while doing the very best I can toward what I prefer." The old man laughed and nodded in approval.

"Most people are grateful when things are good, but you say to be grateful even during tough times. How do you stay grateful when things are not going well, and why would you do that?" I asked the wise old man.

He nodded patiently. "It's easy to be grateful when everything is wonderful, but it is actually more important to express gratitude when you are having a 'tough time.'

How do I stay grateful during tough times? Practice and perception. You see, a 'tough time' is relative. A 'tough time' does not only apply to extreme circumstances like losing your job or suffering a loss in your family. Even trivial things like being stuck in traffic when there is a bad accident can be considered a 'tough time.' It is perfectly normal to be upset over small issues like that, but it is also important to be grateful that you weren't in the accident that caused the traffic jam. You can be grateful for the opportunity to practice gratitude when little things like that happen so that you are well practiced when something even worse happens. There is always something you can be grateful for, and you can never practice too much gratitude."

"How often do you practice gratitude? I hear that many self-improvement gurus recommend practicing gratitude daily," I asked, and the old man laughed.

"Once a day is good to start with if you've never done 'gratitude practice,' and you can work your way to at least twice a day. I like to write down five different things I am grateful for. I might also say them out loud first thing every morning and evening, and also moment to moment, all day, multiple times a day," the old man answered.

"You express five different reasons to be grateful twice a day? That's a lot of gratitude! So you are grateful for every meal? Do you express the same gratitude every time?"

"Yes and no. For example, you can have the same gratitude for every meal, for waking up in the morning, and for being able to go to sleep and rest. But I am also grateful for the warmth and brightness of the sunny day, for the cooler temperature when it's cloudy, for the rain that's good for the trees, for the beautiful memories that I have made with my late wife, for getting laid off from my jobs twice in three years, which inspired me to start this business, for my childhood cancer, which inspired me to live a healthier life, and for many other things. There is always something to be grateful for if you look even just a little bit."

"So, you really believe in the benefit of expressing lots of gratitude? When did you start practicing gratitude?" I asked the old man.

"I don't just believe; I experienced firsthand the benefit of gratitude. I started practicing gratitude at fourteen years of age when I was going through cancer treatment, long before everyone else spoke of practicing it. At the beginning of the treatment, endless pain and frequent hospitalization made me miserable and anxious. One day, a volunteer talked my mom and me into practicing gratitude with her. Back then, I couldn't even be grateful that I was alive because I was so miserable, but I could be grateful that my parents were alive and that my mom was by my side every day. Then I was grateful that I didn't have to do chores or shovel snow, because it was wintertime. Then I was grateful that every time I was in a good enough mood, my older brother would share his new big-boy toys and tricks with me, and a couple of times even let me hang out with his friends. Thinking about these things made me happier, put me in a better mood, and helped me minimize my feelings of anxiety and depression. I also felt less of the nausea from chemotherapy and pain from the cancer. Once I got better, I could go home, and if I stayed well, I could stay home. So, I kept looking for something to be happy about. The next year of treatment flew by, and years later the doctors said that I beat the cancer because I tolerated the treatment so well. If I hadn't learned to practice gratitude, I doubt my treatment would have gone as smoothly."

The old man seemed to be lost in his thoughts for a moment, then he continued. "Nowadays, there are studies that can explain the physical, psychological, and emotional benefits of gratitude. Expressing gratitude reduces inflammation in our body. It also stimulates our hypothalamus, the controller of our appetite and our sleep, so that we can sleep better and have a better appetite. Practicing gratitude also causes the release of dopamine, our feel-good hormone. The increase in our dopamine makes us feel less pain, lowers our heart rate and blood pressure, lessens our anxiety and depression, and helps us to relax. All these benefits put us in a better mood. Overall, this improves our attitudes and our ability to focus. When we can think clearly and focus more, we get more things done, seize more opportunities, and see more things to be grateful about. When we are more pleasant, people like us more, they treat us better, and they become more cooperative. You see, gratitude brings us to live in the Good Circle of Life. If you are going to adopt only one new good practice, adopt the gratitude practice.

Practice gratitude during tough times in addition to good times."

I listened to the wise old man and started my NATO and gratitude practice. To avoid feeling overwhelmed, I started my gratitude practice by writing at least three different reasons to be grateful every night, then I added ten more reasons in the morning and midday, and finally I would add more reasons in the moment-to-moment. I learned the truth that, regardless of life's circumstances, there is always something for which to be grateful. My life has continued to improve rapidly since I started the gratitude practice. The old man has passed away since our conversation, but I am happy and grateful that I had ample opportunity to learn from him. I am grateful that his teaching and gratitude practice has helped me in my life. Now that I help others through gratitude and NATO practice, his teaching continues to help many other people. The gratitude practice indeed brings to life the Good Circle of Life.

Circle of Laughter

What is the favorite drink of a girl named Jasmin Bailey? Jasmine tea with Bailey's Irish cream.

Our fifth tool for being a person with forward-fortitude is to practice humor and have fun with our everyday lives.

It might seem antagonistic to have fun and laugh when our lives are disintegrating right before our very eyes. However, we want to remember that laughing carries many physiological and emotional benefits. Emotionally, laughing improves our mood. We can be happy and laugh, or we can laugh and be happy. Even when we are in the dark valley of our lives, we want to choose to seek fun and laughter at every opportunity.

Physiologically, laughing increases the production of immunoglobulin A and the activation of our natural killer cells and T lymphocytes, all of which help us to have a better immune system.

Laughing also decreases the production of our cortisol, which is our stress hormone, while causing the release of endorphin, our feel-good hormone. The combination of having more endorphins with less cortisol helps to keep our heart rate and blood pressure lower, and we feel more relaxed. When we can stay calm, we will be able to think more clearly about what we might be able to do in order to alleviate our circumstances.

We also want to remember that as dire as our circumstance might seem to us, they are just circumstances. "Circumstance" comes from the Latin words *circum* (meaning "around") and *stare* ("to stand"). When we are experiencing circumstances, we are standing at one spot in our circle of life. We happen to be at a dark spot at this moment, but our circle of life keeps on moving. If we don't give up, we will be in the next brighter part of the circle of our life.

Just as Og Mandino says:

"I will laugh at the world. And how can I laugh when confronted with man or deed which offends me so as to bring forth my tears or my curses? Four words: This too shall pass. I will laugh at the world. For all worldly things shall indeed pass. When I am heavy with heartache, I shall console myself that this too shall pass; when I am puffed with success, I shall warn myself that this too shall pass. And with my laughter, all things will be reduced to their proper size. I will laugh at my failures, and they will vanish in the cloud of new dreams; I will laugh at my successes, and they will shrink to their true value. I will laugh at the world."[12]

For some of us feel as if we had fallen into the dark valley of life a long time ago and are still trapped to this day. The most common reason for this is that we need a different map for navigating ourselves through and beyond our grief.

Some of us feel as if we have been in the dark valley of our lives for as long as we can remember. If we feel this way, we want to explore the possibility that we might have unknowingly been wearing a pair of sunglasses that darkens everything we see. Many people who continuously wear spectacles can become unaware that their glasses are on them; they easily forget that they are wearing a pair of glasses because they are so accustomed to the glasses. This phenomenon can occur metaphorically in our lives as well. If everything in our lives seems to be dark for the longest time, perhaps we will want to explore the possibility of unknowingly wearing sunglasses. To see our lives differently, perhaps we should try wearing a lighter-colored pair of glasses.

It is our choice to push our internal pause button when we notice that we are having disempowering thoughts or undesirable emotions, to decide that we are going to smile instead of swear, to dance in the rain, to laugh and become happy, and to be masters of our thoughts and emotions. What can you do to infuse laughter and fun into your life this week, regardless of your circumstances?

By the way: laughter has been associated with asthma attacks, exacerbation of back/neck problems, and death. Please consult your physician if you have any medical condition for which laughter might be harmful.

Painting and Marching in Bubble Baths

Our sixth tool for being a person with forward-fortitude is to practice truly loving ourselves.

Truly loving ourselves is not being selfish or even self-centered because it is actually good for the people around us. Have you ever been in a commercial plane where the pilot advised you to put your own oxygen mask on first before trying to help others? This is because if we ourselves become asphyxiated, not only will we not be able to help the other passengers, we will become a burden to other people.

Have you ever read, heard about, or perhaps personally known people who have transformed their heartbreak into something that has helped many other people in addition to helping themselves? The first thing they did was to work on healing their broken heart; by doing this, they discovered something that was good for themselves and for others. Have you ever met someone who was so depressed, overwhelmed, or angry that their distress made you feel uncomfortable? This is because everything is energy (Einstein), and we can feel and be affected by the other person's energy even without them saying a word. The same goes the other way: others can feel our energy if we are in emotional pain but try to put on a brave face and pretend that we are fine. Other people can feel if we are overwhelmed or annoyed, and they can be affected by the emotional state that we are trying to hide. Keeping all these things in mind, it is clear that loving ourselves is serving, not selfish.

There are three components of loving ourselves: expression, kind respect, and action.

The first component is to express.

Have you ever had a large pimple? For a large pimple to heal completely, we need to allow the content to flow out. If we don't allow the content to clear out, even after the inflammation is resolved, the pimple stays as a hard bump. The best way to allow the content of the pimple to flow out is by gently creating a small hole in it instead of squeezing it. Squeezing a pimple causes more damage to the already irritated tissue and can actually delay and complicate the healing process.

The grief that we experience from our tragedy is like having a large boil or pimple on our emotional hearts, and all our thoughts and feelings associated with our grief are like the contents inside the pimple. Just like with the large pimple, we want to allow these thoughts and feelings to flow out so that they don't become long-term scars, just like an unexpressed pimple. Also, we want to express our thoughts in a smart and safe way. Just as we do not want to squeeze a pimple to make it rupture and create more tissue damage, we do not want to wait in expressing our thoughts and feelings and end up "exploding" at someone we happen to be interacting with and thus creating even more problems in our lives.

One way to express our emotions is through words: by speaking with trusted friends or a counselor, journaling, or even creative writing. However, for some of us, talking about our grief is not a helpful outlet. For some of us, we are either lost in our emotions or we have "numbed" ourselves as a reaction to our trauma, and thus have difficulty expressing our feelings. Even for those who are able to express their emotions through words, there is a part of grief that words cannot touch. If you find that speaking or writing about your grief does not allow you to fully express your grief, you want to find a different way to do it. Some people paint or do some other form of art, some sing in the shower, some exercise, some listen to music, and some dance.

I personally find expressive freestyle dancing helpful in allowing my feelings to flow. Dr. Joe Dispenza says that when we read or hear something, we store it in our mind. When we have an impactful experience, it gets stored at a cellular level. When we move our bodies, such as while we are dancing or exercising, we move our cells and allow the stored, stuck energy to move and flow away more easily. Many scholars have found that music helps us feel much better. This is the reason why freestyle dancing, such as that used in Dance Away Sadness: Move Beyond Your Grief, is helpful in facilitating our emotional expressions to move through and beyond our grief. Whatever you find helpful for you to express your grief and other feelings, please explore it early in your journey. Do not wait until it's too late: start moving now.

The second component of loving ourselves is kind respect.

What is kind respect? Kind respect is like having a friend whom we love and respect greatly. Imagine this friend is now going through a very tough time and misspoke a simple fact or forgot an appointment with you. Would you start saying things like "stupid," or "crazy," or even "how could you?" to your beloved friend for their mistake? Most likely, you would express empathy and love. For some reason, we often do the exact opposite to ourselves. We often speak harshly to ourselves if we catch ourselves doing or saying something that we wish we had not said or done. Let's be our own best friend and express more love to ourselves, just as we would to the friend that we greatly love and respect.

Also, when we respect someone, we listen to them. When we respect ourselves, we listen to our feelings, thoughts, and bodies to discover what we need to heal. For some of us, it might be sleeping more, while for others it might be changing their diet, exploring a different way of thinking, or having more "me" time. Since we love and respect ourselves, we are mindful of what we allow into our bodies and minds. As Og Mandino says:

"And most of all I will love myself ... I will zealously inspect all things which enter my body, my mind, my soul, and my heart ... I will cherish my body with cleanliness and moderation ... my mind ... I will uplift it with the knowledge and wisdom of the ages ... my soul ... I will feed it with meditation and prayer ... my heart ... I will share it, and it will grow and warm the earth."

We must learn to listen to our hearts and bodies and do what we intuitively feel is good for us.

The third component of loving ourselves is action.

We act inwardly and outwardly. Acting inwardly is when we do things that are good for us personally. It is when we dance every night in our living room as I did, just to allow our grief to flow. It is when we start meditating, start a healthier eating regimen, or start listening to more empowering healing messages. Acting inwardly is saying "no" to things that we feel are not life-giving, such as refusing to accompany your single sister on a double-blind date nine months after your marriage had dissolved and taking a bubble bath instead. Many of us are uncomfortable saying no because we want to be nice or we don't want to hurt other people's feelings. However, as we discovered at the start of this section, other people can feel our emotions even without us saying them. If you were to put on a happy face and go on the blind date while you were still in a lot of anguish and pain, the other people in the group would most likely feel it anyway, and now you might actually ruined their time by trying to be brave and pretending to be happy. Let's take the action that is serving all instead, and sometimes that means saying no to something your heart doesn't want you to do. Take the bubble bath instead.

Acting outwardly is doing things that can potentially improve our currently undesirable circumstances, so do them promptly! We do not want to fake a brave or happy face, but we do want to do what we can to feel happy sooner. Often, we wait for circumstances to change in order to be happy even though we could be happy right where we are. I could have waited for my dominant hand to improve before I decided to laugh and be happier, but I decided instead to start finding reasons to smile and laugh, all while waiting at the MRI facility. In many cases, it is changing our thinking and our perception that allows us to see opportunities that we can act on to help us recover from our grief and thrive.

Acting outwardly is taking the steps we can in the very moment they come to us. Unfortunately, many people hesitate to grasp an opportunity, worrying that it might not work out the way they want it to. This hesitation is very understandable, particularly when we are already having a tough time. However, a good opportunity is like a slippery fish: it will be gone, never to return, if we don't grasp it when it comes within reach. Don't wait until all "the ducks are in a row" before you take actions to improve your situation. Do you even have ducks? There is a saying that "even God cannot move a parked car." Release your brake and start driving today. Even if we only drive a mile a day at the start, we will eventually make it to our destination. We will travel from our loss and grief to our new lives one baby step at a time, if need be.

Just to recap, our sixth tool for being a person with forward-fortitude is to practice loving ourselves. We kindly respect ourselves, express our thoughts and feelings, take self-care actions, and take actions that can help us to improve our circumstances. Doing these along with the nine-second move helps us focus on the "what is" and on simplifying our lives. Practicing NATO with gratitude, learning to laugh at ourselves and the world, and having a more empowered perception will help us to move through our troubles with more ease and at a faster pace.

Let's "Cheers"

"When did you start using chopsticks with your left hand?" my mother asked with amusement.

"Since I lost function in my right hand," I laughed in reply. "I can't use chopsticks with my right hand for now, so I trained myself to use my left hand. I have started writing and doing other things with my left hand, too. When my right hand recovers, I'll be ambidextrous, which I think is cool. Let's 'cheers' to me being able to use chopsticks with my left hand!"

The seventh and final tool of being a person with

forward-fortitude is to celebrate genuinely. It might seem strange to you to celebrate while you are having a tough time. However, celebrating is a cheerful practice of gratefulness, which requires us to find something positive in our lives and feel the positivity enough to be cheerful about it. Just as we do not want to fake a happy face, we do not fake cheerfulness. What we do is simply shift our focus to perceiving that the glass does not need to be half empty—it can be refilled if you choose to do so. Until our glass is full of sparkling water, we can be grateful and celebrate our ability to pour sparkling water into it. Just as we celebrate and cheer a baby's first step, we endeavor to focus our minds on the good, no matter how small. We rejoice with every little improvement in our situation, just as when a little butterfly rejoices in its first flight.

REVIEW

1. Unmet hopes are often an overlooked cause of grief. They are as impactful as the tragic event itself—sometimes more so.
2. Practicing forward-fortitude allows us to move through our grief journey with more ease, to recover and thrive faster and more completely.
3. Being able to understand perception is the first skill for forward-fortitude. Is the beach ball blue or red? What about after you step back and take off your dark sunglasses?
4. The nine-second master-move: Notice—Pause—Choose—Decide.

5. Breathe in the simple present to reduce your worries and regrets.
6. NATO with gratitude.
7. Laugh.
8. Self-love = express + kind respect + act.
9. Celebrate.

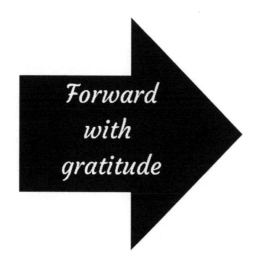

Forward
with
gratitude

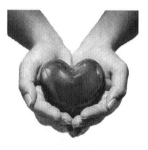

Chapter 5

LITTLE BUTTERFLY

The fifth step for navigating through our disaster and the grief associated with it comes from our fifth finger: our little one. We use our little finger to remind us about the metamorphosis of a beautiful little butterfly that can help keep us strong in our journey. We also use our little fingers to remind us to pay attention to the little things and to look for the little seeds of good throughout the journey that will help us to move through our dark valley and into a better life in a smoother and easier fashion.

LITTLE SEED OF GOLDEN GREEN PLUM

"I don't see how losing my home in the fire could have

any seed of good in it; I don't see any good at all," Mark said over the video call, with discouragement and despair that turned into visible irritation.

"You said you had a garden before the fire burned everything down, and that you had a great big green plum tree that gave you lots of fruits, and that you and your family had fun picnicking under it every summer. Did you grow this green plum tree, the one you called your precious golden green plum tree, from a seed?" I asked Mark.

"Yes, I did. It took almost five years, but then it became a great tree with lots of sweet plums every year since. Why?" Mark answered, still sounding irritated.

"When your green plum was a seed, did that seed look like an actual plum? Or did it actually look like a plum seed with a hard, rough surface and a little sharp pointy end?" I asked Mark. He looked confused for a moment on the video call.

"What do you mean? The plum seed looked like a plum seed. It did not look like the fruit or the tree. Have you never seen a plum seed?"

I nodded and smiled, "Yes, I have seen a plum seed, but I wanted to make sure that your magnificent green plum tree did look like a seed when it was a seed. A simple seed inside of a hard shell with a rough, abrasive surface and one sharp pointy end. Compared to the look of the fruit, it was an ugly seed that, if you tossed it in the trash instead of planting in fertile soil and nurturing it, it would not have become what you call your golden green plum tree. It was your act of planting the seed and nurturing it every day that gave you a very lovely plum tree."

I could see Mark's eyes widen and his face brighten as he nodded slightly, "I got it. The seed of good would not look like the great things that are still coming."

I nodded, "Correct. It usually does not come in a package with a big bow. Usually, you need to find the seed. And just like with a real seed, you need to plant the seed in your life and then nurture it daily until it grows into a plant. Do that with love and trust."

"That's the problem," Mark interrupted. I have a hard time blindly believing that there's good in having everything burned down. And I just can't find the seed of good."

"I understand. I can see how you can't see any seed of good after having everything burn down in the fire," I said gently. "Let me ask you, Mark, what made you believe that the seed of your green plum could grow into a fruitful tree when it was just a little seed?"

Mark frowned slightly. "The plum was different. I had grown another plum tree from seed. It wasn't green, but it was still a plum tree. I know about plants and plum trees and how it would grow. I did what I needed to do for it and then relaxed and gave it time, and the plants always did fine."

"Okay, so you trusted that the seed would grow into a plant even when you could not see anything on the ground yet. You had the knowledge that if you nurtured the seed and sprouted it in a certain way, it would grow into a plant and give you great fruits. You could relax because you knew what you were doing. But people who have never grown a plum tree from a seed, such as myself, might have a tougher time just relaxing and trusting and giving it time, even when they have done everything they needed to have good fruits from a seed. Some people might even have difficulty believing that they can grow a plum seed to the point that it gives lots of great fruits because they don't have the knowledge or experience." I paused to see if Mark could follow my thought process.

He laughed. "I grow real seeds, and you grow abstract ones."

"You have grown physical fruit seeds, and now you can grow nonphysical life seeds too. Since this is new for you, you might find it challenging to believe that there is a seed of greater good within your tragedy. However, you do know people who have done that well, just as I know people who have grown and harvested fruits from seeds that they have grown. If they can do it, I can do it too, particularly if I have their guidance. If I and many others can thrive from our tragedies, you can too, and it'll be a lot easier and faster if you continue following and trusting your guide."

Mark smiled. "Okay. I trust you, but I still can't find any seeds of good." I was glad to see that Mark could at least smile again.

"Well, sometimes we cannot see it right away because what we can see is very much influenced by our awareness and state of mind. That's why we want to allow for some quiet time for doing the 'Finding Seeds of Good' exercise, and doing it more than once, even if we find some good the first time we do it. How many times have you done the exercise, and how much quiet time did you put into doing it each time?"

I could see over the video that Mark lowered his gaze and paused before he said, "Well, I did it once for a few minutes. I really couldn't believe that there was any seed of good in this tragedy," he said defiantly. "But I trust you and your knowledge and experience, and you really believe that there's a seed of greater good, so I'll do the game over again."

An intuition came to me. "You said that the plum tree was a big tree. Is it still standing? Have you looked at it closely since the fire?"

"It's all charred but still standing. No, I have not looked at it closely. I can't bear looking at that burned-down place for too long." Mark's face expressed despair as he spoke.

"I'm so sorry it's been so painful, Mark. I'm sending virtual hugs to you. Please feel my arms surround you and envelop you with love, good energy, and strength. I was asking if you have looked at your green plum tree closely to see if the core is still alive. I know some trees can get burned on the outside, but the insides stay alive and they can recover. Would you mind checking out the core of your green plum tree?"

Mark looked hesitant. "It looked pretty charred, and all the leaves and branches were burned. I strongly doubt it is still alive. Not impossible, but extremely unlikely." I was glad Mark said it was not impossible for his tree to still be alive.

"Okay, so it's improbable but not impossible. Would you consider checking out that tree, please? If you decide that you are going to look closely at the tree, perhaps you can do it much sooner, perhaps even today if you want to?"

My phone rang a few hours later. It was Mark, exhilarated. "You're not gonna believe this. All the trees here burned and died, except the green plum tree. My golden green plum tree is still alive; the core is still alive. I can hardly believe it. My prized possession, my precious golden green plum tree, is still alive. This is a good sign. There is hope. Thank you. Thank you for having me check it. I can nurture it back to health with lots of love; it'll have great fruits again and my family and I can create new great memories picnicking under it again. Thank you for believing that there's hope and not giving up when I couldn't believe it. Thank you!"

Napoleon Hill said, "Every adversity, every heartbreak, every failure carries in it the seed of an equal or greater benefit." However, it can be challenging for some of us to find this seed of greater good, for it is usually hidden in the ashes of our traumatic events. For others, it is challenging even to believe that there is a benefit waiting to emerge from our disaster. If you cannot believe that there is good coming from your tragedy, please know that you don't have to believe anything. You just need to be open-minded enough to take the next step to help you recover from your grief and thrive. Follow the footsteps of many others by developing the need to thrive. To help you find this seed of greater benefit from your experience, I have developed a system: the "Finding Seeds of Good" exercise that is described in the Appendix. Once we find a seed of possible good, we want to plant it in the fertile soil of our open mind and heart, and nurture it daily the best we can. Just as we do not expect a plum seed to grow into a tree and start producing fruit in two months, we might not see the sweet fruits of our adversity right away. However, with proper care and fertilizing, our plum seed might start producing sweet fruits faster than you expect. This is the same with our seed of greater goods. If we consistently and relentlessly do what it takes to thrive, we will move through our dark valley and thrive with ease.

LITTLE MESSY BUTTERFLY AND PHOENIX

My phone rang, waking me from my deep sleep. I looked at the clock; it was 11:15 at night. It was Fawn calling. She had been feeling more sadness recently as she approached what would have been the first birthday of her unborn son. "Hi, Fawn. Is everything okay?" I asked with concern, as it was unlike her to call late at night.

"I just dreamed of Archie," Fawn said with a shaky voice. Archie was the name Fawn gave to the son she had miscarried.

"Oh! How was Archie in your dream? How are you?"
I asked.

I could hear Fawn take a deep breath. "I'm sad he is
not here. I dreamed that he was older, like five or six years
old. We were playing in a flower field. He was very happy
as he played in the field. Then a butterfly landed on his
hand and he gave the butterfly to me. He said, 'Mommy,
it's your butterfly, I'm bringing you your butterfly.' I took
the butterfly and Archie skipped and hopped into the
flower field, laughing happily until he vanished. I can still
hear him laugh." Fawn's voice faltered.

"So, he was happy in your dream and he gave you a
butterfly. How does that make you feel?" I asked carefully.

Fawn took a little time before she answered, "I am
sad Archie is not here, and I'm confused and scared."

"Why are you scared?" I asked, wondering what
could scare Fawn.

I could hear Fawn fully exhale before she said, "I'm
scared because I don't know why this happened to me. I
have read about people going through metamorphosis,
though not physically. I think Archie was implying that I
am too: I am going through a metamorphosis. But why?
What am I supposed to do or become? And why me?"

My mind went back to June 19, 2013. My heart was
so broken that I had shortness of breath, and I felt like I
needed to vomit. Why? Why did all these miseries happen
one after another within the last two years? Just when I
thought that things were getting better, Roscoe died. He
was my only friend and my guardian angel, and he died

suddenly. It felt like someone had ripped open a scab that was just forming over the wound from my divorce. To make matters worse, Bootsie died only nine days after Roscoe. She was fine one day and gone the next. She was my last cat. It felt like someone had poured acid over my open wound. I thought I had made it through the two years of misery, but the tragedies continued to pile up. Why did I have to go through two years of dark nights only to be squeezed again just when I thought I could see the light?

The answer was that I was undergoing a metamorphosis from the caterpillar version of myself to the butterfly version. The word "metamorphosis" comes from the Latin word *metamorphoun*, which means to transform or change shape. According to the Google online dictionary, metamorphosis is a change of the form or nature of a thing or person into something completely different. Many of us know that a caterpillar must go through a metamorphosis in order to become a butterfly. Few people, however, are aware that the newly formed butterfly has to go through a second squeezing as it works its way out of the pupae. During this phase of second squeezing, the new butterfly develops its wings, gets rid of excess fluid that would only weigh it down, and builds muscle strength to be able to fly. If the newly formed butterfly does not work its muscles, it will not be able to fly and will soon die.

Sometimes, we humans go through metamorphosis too, though not physically. Often, our adversities occur to help us transform into more empowered versions of ourselves. Unfortunately, we sometimes make this process longer and more painful than it already is. A caterpillar will keep going through the liquefying process of its body without pausing or giving up. On the other hand, we humans, because of our ability to choose, often resist this unpleasant process.

Some of us give up entirely and become bitter instead of better, which goes further to killing our livelihood even if we are still alive physically. Most of us keep going through our adversities one after another without any resistance. It is natural for us to want to resist something that is unpleasant. Unfortunately, resisting only creates friction, and friction slows things down. When we resist our adversities, we do not make them go away. Instead, it takes a lot longer for us to move through the process. What we want to endeavor is to go through the process with as little resistance as we can, learn from the experience, and find the seed of greater good as fast as we possibly can.

We endeavor because, unlike the caterpillar and the upcoming butterfly, our metamorphosis will likely be imperfect. Metamorphosis is a messy process. Physically, if we were to open a pupa during the early stage of its metamorphosis, we would find a mess of gooey liquid and chunks of digested caterpillar body. Even after the new butterfly has been formed, everything inside the chrysalis is still messy and cramped together. When we undergo our metamorphosis, our lives often look messy, but this is very normal.

Moving through metamorphosis is not a linear

process. As we walk through the dark valleys of our lives, we might trip, get sidetracked, fall backward, get discouraged, or suffer any other imaginable cause of delay. This is normal. Having expert guidance will help to minimize these additional problems, but even with expert guidance, we still might feel like everything has become a mess. Indeed, everything is a mess. It is normal and natural for everything to be a mess, and we feel like a mess when we are moving through our transformation. Just endeavor not to resist the mess, or pause it, or give up during our metamorphosis. Hold on one more day and keep taking steps forward even if you have to crawl. Remember not to give up when you receive a second "big squeeze," which you might experience toward the end of your metamorphosis. The more we exercise our flying muscles, the stronger, higher, and further we can fly to bring good to ourselves and others.

Three years had passed since the night Fawn called me to tell me about her dream of her unborn son when I got another call from her. Fawn decided to change her vocation to become a grief coach, write a book, and start an online support group that provides emotional support for women who either had a miscarriage or had to give up their child after birth. "Would you please help me with the online group?"

I told her I would. Fawn thanked me. "Oh, and we talked about metamorphosis earlier in my journey. What about the phoenix?" she asked.

"I am not sure what you are asking," I said.

Fawn chuckled, "I recently read about phoenix rising: the process in which a phoenix burns itself into ashes and a new one comes up in its place. What makes you think I had a metamorphosis instead of a phoenix experience?"

I thought about it, "I honestly don't know why I chose to tell you about metamorphosis instead of phoenix rising when I was trying to illustrate transformation to you. I guess the results are the same in the end. Whichever transformation path we go through, at the end, all of our tragedies and grief make us more empowered, and benefit others as well."

As Shakespeare says, "Sweet are the uses of adversity."

Lighten Up

Have you ever tried to run with a heavy rock-filled backpack on your back? If you have, you know the heavy backpack will slow you down significantly. Imagine if a caterpillar were to try to fly—the wings of a butterfly would have difficulty supporting the body that is much heavier than its butterfly body. This is the same reason small planes have weight limitations. For a butterfly to be able to fly gracefully, it needs to let go of all the excess tissue and fluid.

This is the same as when we undergo a nonphysical metamorphosis. For the butterfly version of us to be able to fly easily and gracefully, we need to be able to let go of certain things that are no longer serving us well. These things could even be tangible, such as all the extra junk we have in our storage units.

Things to let go of often include intangible matters as well. These could be relationships that have become more destructive than beneficial. These could be heavy feelings we still carry from our past, whether from our recent tragedies or beyond, that still wake us up in the middle of the night, and should be let go. Letting go of any resentments, residual anger, blame, guilt, and shame is crucial for us to be able to transition into the butterfly version of ourselves. Please revisit the sections on "Hung by a String of Gs" and "The F Word" if there is any residual anger, shame, or guilt that you can let go of. Once we have shed our unnecessary excess weight, we will be able to fly fully into the butterfly version of ourselves.

THE LITTLE ANT THAT COULD

Our metamorphosis typically is not linear, nor is it an easy process. One thing that can help ease our journey today is to look for and cherish the little things that are still good in our lives. Perhaps it is a particularly beautiful full moon, or an extra-friendly grocery clerk, or a solo wildflower that grew from a crack in the sidewalk, or a determined little ant moving a crumb of bread because it believed it could.

Noticing and cherishing little things helps us to heal our broken hearts. Emotionally and physically, doing so helps us to become calmer and feel better. We need to be at a certain level of calmness in order to be able to notice little things in life. When we consciously choose to pay attention to the little things, we direct our nervous system to calm down. When we are calmer, we tend to breathe slower and deeper, and thus take in more oxygen. The increase in our oxygenation helps us to feel much better, more energized, and even more peaceful. Also, when we notice little things that we choose to cherish, we take our attention away from the pain that we might be feeling. When we are not focusing on something, we will notice it less often. When we are focused on the beauty of life, we will feel less of the pain.

In addition to noticing the little things that are still good, doing good things for others, no matter how small, is also very beneficial. Imagine that you are standing at the grocery line and you notice that the purple highlight on the checkout clerk matches her glasses frame perfectly and you compliment her. Would that make her feel happy and possibly be friendlier to you? Almost certainly. Would being able to compliment someone on such subtle little things make you feel better? Very likely. Would her friendliness as a result of your no-cost small gesture make you feel better too? Most likely. Often, the effect of a nice little gesture is much bigger than most of us actually realize. A good little thing is indeed the source of a great big thing. What little thing could you cherish or do today?

CLOSING WORDS

Wabi-Sabi Dream

The Japanese have a philosophy called *wabi-sabi* that involves finding beauty in imperfection. One expression of wabi-sabi is to break a vase and put the pieces back together. Often, the pieces do not fit perfectly and this allows light into the rebuilt vase. The light will create a beautiful pattern in the vase, one that is only possible because the vase was rebuilt imperfectly.

More often than not, we want things in our lives to go perfectly. We want our body, our home, our hair, our title, the way we do things, and the way others do or say things to be perfect according to the illusion that we have created in our minds. It is an illusion that is very often influenced by what society deems as "perfect."

For the longest time, I despised my thick calves so much that I would not wear a skirt. I hated them because in my younger years, I compared myself to magazine pictures of pencil-thin models with very slim legs. Early in my metamorphosis, I started to do freestyle dancing in order to release the part of grief that words could not touch. I started by dancing in my bedroom. As I healed, I created Dance Away Sadness: Move Beyond Your Grief to help others heal as well. I have also learned to enjoy and benefit from hiking. Having legs with big, strong muscles allows me to be able to dance and hike for a long time without my legs becoming tired. As a bonus, my legs fit perfectly in knee-high boots, which match perfectly with the skirts I now love to wear. I am so very grateful for my beautiful legs. They are still imperfect now, but at the same time, they have always been perfect for me.

So, what is perfection? Perfection is an illusion, a

goal that we can never attain for long. There is nothing perfect in life. Our journeys through life, whether good or bad, are not meant to be perfect. In striving for perfection, we want to endeavor to find beauty in the imperfection of ourselves and our lives. We want to choose to let go of the illusion that we can have perfection.

To Do or Not to Do: It Is Your Choice

I invite you to choose to endeavor in letting go of perfection, in looking for the seed of good and noticing and cherishing the little things at the same time, in having a two-thumbs-up attitude as your tears flow, and in practicing the nine-second master-move alongside NATO with gratitude. I invite you to choose these things regardless of what has happened in your life: "That was then, this is now."[9] Choose to endeavor for the next chapters in your book of life to be chapters of recovery and triumph. We will do our best, but we know we will not do it perfectly. I invite you to choose not only to recover, but to thrive as well—because it is your only choice. As the Grief Recovery Institute says, you need to take at least one percent responsibility: the responsibility of wanting to recover and transform your failure and tragedies into triumphs and joyful living. I bring the water to you, but I cannot and will not make you drink it.

I hope you join me in choosing to find and plant the seeds of greater good. I am very excited to share with you that very recently, my right hand and arm recovered completely, and I am now living with even better health.

I know that no matter what the future brings, there are seeds of greater good in it for all.

REVIEW

1. There is a seed of good even in this adversity. Use the "Finding Seeds of Good" exercise to find and plant the seed of good and burn the rest away.
2. You don't have to believe. You only need to be open-minded.
3. Every seed needs to be planted and nurtured before you can harvest the fruit.
4. Metamorphosis often requires another struggle before you can fly.
5. Metamorphosis is a messy process.
6. Wabi-sabi.
7. It is your choice.

I am very sorry if you and/or your loved one has had to go through the dark valley of life. Please feel my arms surround you, enveloping you with love and strength for your journey.

I am here for you; *you are not alone.*

> With love, gratitude, and warmest regards,
> Birgitte Tan

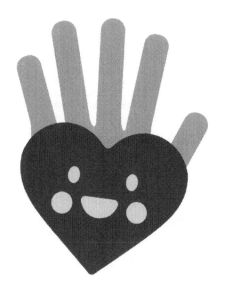

REFERENCES

1. The Grief Recovery Method. (n.d.). Retrieved October 1, 2019, from https://www.griefrecoverymethod.com/.

2. J. Murube, "Basal, Reflex, and Psycho-Emotional Tears," *Ocular Surface* 7, no. 2 (April 2009): 60—6.

3. Reena Mukamal, "All About Emotional Tears," American Academy of Ophthalmology, accessed January 21, 2020, https://www.aao.org/eye-health/tips-prevention/all-about-emotional-tears/.

4. A. Skorucak, "The Science of Tears," retrieved October 1, 2019, www.ScienceIQ.com.

5. Chen Feisong and Gai Guozhong, *Hand Reflexology & Acupressure: A Natural Way to Health through Traditional Chinese Medicine* (New York, NY: Better Link Press, 2019), 15—25.

6. Maxwell Maltz, *The Magic Power of Self-Image Psychology: The New Way to a Bright, Full Life* (New York, NY: Pocket Books, 1970), 1—12.

7. Eve Caligor, Kenneth Levy, and Frank Yeomans, "Narcissistic Personality Disorder: Diagnostic and Clinical Challenges," *American Journal of Psychiatry* 172, no. 5 (May 2015): 415—8.

8. R. Friedman, The Grief Recovery Institute (Bend, OR), personal communication.

9. M. Morrissey, personal communication.

10. R. Jerath, J. W. Edry, V. A. Barnes, and V. Jerath, "Physiology of Long Pranayamic Breathing: Neural Respiratory Elements May Provide a Mechanism that Explains How Slow, Deep Breathing Shifts the Autonomic Nervous System," *Medical Hypotheses* 67, no. 3 (2006): 566—71.

11. Henry Thoreau, "Economy," in *Walden* (London, UK: CRW Publishing Limited, 1854), 7—86.

12. Og Mandino, "The Scroll Marked VII," in *The Greatest Salesman in the World* (Hollywood, FL: Frederick Fell Publisher, 1968), 83—7.

APPENDIX

DEEP BREATHING TECHNIQUE

If possible, sit with your back straight or lie down on a firm surface.

Curl your tongue such that the tip of your tongue touches the roof of your mouth behind the inside of your upper teeth (unless you are physically unable to do this). Please keep the tip of your tongue connected to the roof of your mouth throughout inhalation and while briefly holding your breath.[13]

You do not need to exhale through your mouth for this deep breathing exercise. If you prefer to exhale through your mouth, you can temporarily disconnect the tip of your tongue from the roof of your mouth to exhale. Please reconnect them prior to holding your breath briefly and inhaling again.

Allow your hands to relax on your lap or by your side. Open your hands such that they are not in a fist position.

Allow your legs and feet to rest in a comfortable position, but it is best not to cross them.

Close your eyes if it is safe to do so.

Allow your body to relax as much as you can while keeping your spine straight.

1) Start by exhaling fully.

2) With the tip of your tongue touching the roof of your mouth behind your upper teeth, inhale deeply, holding the breath for a count of three. Exhale fully and hold the exhale for a slow count of three.

3) Inhale deeply again, this time feeling grateful that you do not need a machine to help you breathe. Hold your breath for a count of three, exhale fully and completely. Hold your breath for a count of three.

4) Take another deep, deep breath and hold for a count of three. Release completely with a long, full exhale, allowing your shoulders to lower and relax. Hold for a count of three.

5) Keeping the tip of your tongue on the roof of your mouth behind your upper teeth, inhale another deep, deep breath of good, healing energy. Hold for a count of three, then exhale completely while allowing the rest of your body to relax along with your shoulders. Hold for a count of three.

6) Inhale another deep, deep breath of good healing

energy and send the energy to your mind, holding for a count of three. Release with a long, full exhale while allowing your mind to open and the exhaled breath to take any stress, worry, doubt, and anxiety far, far away into the clouds. Hold for a count of three.

7) Inhale another deep, deep breath of good, healing energy and infinite love. Send the energy and love to your heart and hold for a count of three. Release a long, full exhale completely, while allowing your heart to open and the exhaled breath to take any stress, sadness, fear, and pain far, far away into the clouds. Hold for a count of three.

8) Inhale another deep, deep breath of good healing energy and infinite love, while feeling grateful for being able to do deep breathing. Send the healing energy to your mind and heart and hold for a count of three. Release with a long, full exhale while allowing the exhaled breath to take away any thoughts or feelings that are still weighing you down. Hold for a count of three.

9) Take a normal breath in with a big smile. Exhale normally with an even bigger smile if possible.

DISCLAIMER: Please consult your physician prior to starting any exercise, including this deep breathing exercise. Performing any exercises mentioned in this book implies that you release Birgitte P. Tan and Birgitte Tan LLC of any liability in the aforementioned regard.

FINDING SEEDS OF
GOOD EXERCISE

Find some quiet time and space, then list your adversities and apparent and potential goods.

Your adversities: troubles, unpleasant feelings, disempowering thoughts	Apparent and potential lessons and good from your adversities
Example: I am unable to do my daily tasks due to loss of function in my dominant hand.	Apparent good and lessons: I have learned to be grateful for simple things, such as being able to hold my toothbrush and brush my teeth with my non-dominant hand.
Example: I am unable to do my daily tasks due to loss of function in my dominant hand.	Potential good: This adversity has inspired me to write this book, which will hopefully benefit other people.

Your adversity:	Apparent or potential lessons/ good:

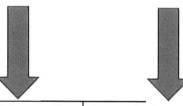

After you pick out all the possible seeds of good, toss your leftover adversities into a fire in your mind. See the fire burn away your adversities. As you watch the smoke from the fire dissipate into the sky, you see that your problems dissipate with the smoke. You have picked out all the seeds of good; now the rest of your unpleasant feelings, disempowering thoughts, troubles, and problems dissipate with the smoke, never to return. You feel more peace and ease.	As you look at your potential seeds of good, sort them. Some lessons and potential seeds of good you will want to keep in the storage of your mind. Other seeds of good are to be planted immediately in your mind and heart. Nourish and grow the seeds of good you are planting. Harvest the good fruits from your circumstances and thrive joyfully.

I recommend you do this exercise in a calm and relaxed state at least three times in the next 30 days.

DISCLAIMER AND
CRISIS LINES

Please be advised that any recommendation in this book is NOT medical, psychiatric, or psychological advice, and NOT a substitute for medical, psychiatric, or psychological care. Your purchasing this book implies that you release Birgitte P. Tan DVM and Birgitte Tan LLC of any liability in the aforementioned regards.

If you are severely overwhelmed by your grief and/or condition and feel suicidal, or know someone who is, please immediately call:

> **In the United States: National Suicide Hotline, 1-800-273-8255 (1-800-273-TALK)**
>
> **In Canada: Crisis Service Canada, 1-833-456-4566**
>
> If someone is in immediate danger of suicide in the United States or Canada, please call 911
>
> Other countries: please call your country's emergency/crisis line.

If you are under the care of a physician or therapist and you feel suicidal, please call your medical professional right away.

If you or someone you know is in a life-threatening situation, please call your country's crisis line immediately.

CONTACT INFORMATION AND ADDITIONAL RESOURCES

CONTACT INFORMATION

Email: support@BirgitteTan.com

Website: http://fromgrievingtojoyfulliving.com/

Telephone: (805) 864-2002

Facebook: https://www.facebook.com/FromGrievingTo JoyfulLiving/

YouTube: https://www.youtube.com/channel/UCrQwB7 7fT2OviUkShdVYBqw/featured

Mailing address:

> The 5-Fingers Method
> 3835 E Thousand Oaks Blvd # 268
> Westlake Village, CA 91362
> USA

ADDITIONAL RESOURCES

I invite you to visit the "From Grieving to Joyful Living" website, Facebook page, and YouTube channel for:

Weekly peace of mind tips

Video example of deep breathing meditation

Guided meditations with Dr. Birgitte Tan

Video example of Dance Away Sadness: Move Beyond Your Grief

Printable gratitude book with healing inspirational quotes

Link to the From Grieving to Joyful Living gratitude group

Short daily teachings and inspiration

Links to other useful resources

Opportunities from Dr. Birgitte Tan

ABOUT ICCC
(International Childhood Cancer Charity)

Ida* dreamed of becoming a pediatric nurse. She felt happy when she could help the younger kids in her sub-Saharan village feel better and happier. Unfortunately, Ida was diagnosed with surgically curable liver cancer when she was eleven. Curable—except for those who could not afford surgery, such as Ida and her family. After seven long years of agony, Ida died one week before her eighteenth birthday. Not only did Ida lose her life, and her family their precious daughter/granddaughter/sister/cousin—but we all lost a beautiful person who could have offered love and healing to others, had her family been able to afford the surgery.

ICCC is here to help children like Ida. ICCC's mission is to help impoverished children with cancer worldwide to heal both physically and emotionally. ICCC provides resources, funding, education, and coaching programs for each child and their parents, to help them beat cancer and thrive with ease and joy.

Please join ICCC and help more light to shine forth onto humanity.

100% of the proceeds from the sale of this book will be donated to the International Childhood Cancer Charity, a 501(c)(3) organization.

* Name has been changed to protect privacy.

Made in the USA
San Bernardino, CA
01 July 2020